girlology

A Girl's Guide to Stuff That Matters

girlology

A Girl's Guide to Stuff* That Matters

*Relationships, body talk & girl power!

Melisa Holmes, M.D.

&

Patricia Hutchison, M.D.

Health Communications, Inc.
Deerfield Beach, Florida
www.hcibooks.com

Library of Congress Cataloging-in-Publication Data

Homes, Melisa.
    Girlology : a girl's guide to stuff that matters : relationships, bodytalk & girl power / Melisa Holmes & Patricia Hutchison.
      p. cm.
    ISBN-13: 978-0-7573-0295-4
    ISBN-10: 0-7573-0295-5
    1. Girls—Life skills guides.   2. Girls—Psychology.   3. Girls—Conduct of life.
I. Hutchison, Patricia.   II. Title.

HQ777.H664 2005
646.7'0082—dc22

2005052506

Publisher: Health Communications, Inc.
           3201 S.W. 15th Street
           Deerfield Beach, FL 33442-8190

R-11-06

Cover and Inside design by Larissa Hise Henoch
Cover illustration and Inside art by Emily Eldridge
Inside Illustration also by Kevin Stawieray and Melisa Holmes
Inside book formatting by Dawn Von Strolley Grove

Contents

PART ONE

Stuck in the Middle

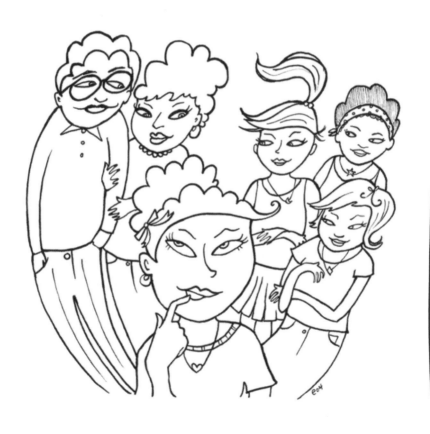

Why Me? Why Now?

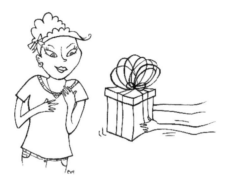

Spin, spin, spin. If you are a preteen or teen girl, we bet that's what your head is doing right now!

You are probably whirling in a sea of mysterious body changes, relationship blowups and confusing information. At school and with friends, you hear chatter about periods, gossip about boyfriends and whispers about sex.

And you are probably bursting with questions. What is all this hair in weird places? Exactly how does sex happen, and why would *anyone* want to do *that*? Do I use the nasty words I see on the bathroom wall to talk about sex? What's this stuff in my underwear? What's up with my friends? Why do we fight and then make up all the time now? How do you tell the difference between a "boyfriend" and a friend who's a boy? How about love and lust? And why don't my parents get it anymore?

Guess what? **There's nothing wrong with having questions or wanting to know more—especially when it comes to your body, sex and relationships.** All those crazy and confusing questions . . . they're normal! And you probably are, too! (Do we hear a big sigh of relief?)

Girlhood Is a Gift!

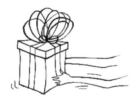

You're a girl. And you are made in an amazing and wonderful way. Because you are a girl, some things are going to happen *to you:* breasts, hips, pimples, periods, crushes on guys, fights with girlfriends, parents who don't get it. You have no choice; they will happen! You are turning into a young woman, and your body and your brain are making these changes because you are developing sexually. So doesn't it make sense that this is the time in your life to learn about these things?

Some things are *guaranteed* to happen. But there are other girl things you can *make choices* about—how you take care of your "new" body, how you use your newfound sex appeal, when you will kiss a guy or how you talk about sex to your parents. **Even though there are a lot of things happening to you that are out of your control, it's good to know that there are a lot of other things that you *can* control.**

Girlology is going to help you open up your girlhood like a gift. We'll rip off the wrapping paper, explore the mysteries inside, learn facts about "all things girl" and help you gain the confidence you need to decide what kind of girl you want to be.

So, What Is **Girlology**?

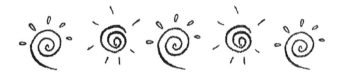

Before we dive in, let's first tell you what *Girlology* is *not:*

- *Girlology* is not a sex talk like you get at school.
- It's not a science lesson.
- It's not like a lecture from your parents.

All those things can be good, but they are not *Girlology.* **Girlology is different.**

Girlology was written by two female doctors who also happen to be mothers of daughters; one of us is a pediatrician (a doctor for children and teenagers up to about 18 years old) and the other is an obstetrician/ gynecologist (fancy words for a doctor who specializes in delivering babies and taking care of girls' and women's body parts that are involved in making babies). Both of us take care of lots of teens who are developing sexually. That means every day we talk to girls thinking about sex . . . avoiding sex . . . having sex . . . confused about sex . . . scared to death about consequences of sex. . . . You name it, we've seen it and talked about it.

We think girls are smart, unique, brave and strong, and we want you to have information that will let all that good stuff shine through!

As doctors, we see girls every day who have the same questions you do. And we see lots of girls and even women who have gotten some *really* wrong answers! No, your period will not stop when you go swimming. Yes, you can get pregnant the first time you have sex. No, you are not gay if you look at a naked girl in the locker room. *Girlology* **is about giving you the straight,** *true* **facts about your body.**

We also treat patients who have made healthy decisions about sex and relationships and others who aren't so happy with the decisions they've made. We want *you* to be happy with the decisions *you* make! *Girlology* is about helping you figure out what's important to you so that you can make decisions you will be pleased with for a long, long, long time.

Girlology is about helping you figure out a lot of things that matter— your body, your relationships and sex. It may sound scary but it's not. *Girlology* is about periods and body parts "down there." It will help you decide how you feel about sex and sexual things. It will help you under-

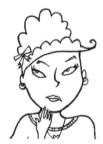

stand guys and learn how to speak up for yourself. It will help you talk to parents and other adults and gain their trust. *Girlology* will also teach you how to understand your friends' and family's values and decide what is important to you. All in all, it's about gaining the confidence you need to develop a special type of "Girl Power!"

We've Got Girl **Power**!

Every school has them: girls who have a special sort of Girl Power. We bet you could name a girl right now who has it. **She's the one other girls trust with secrets, guys respect and teachers count on.**

She may not be the prettiest or most popular, but you can't miss her. She talks, thinks and acts in a way that shows everyone she's confident in who she is and the choices she makes. She's just plain different, but it's a *good* kind of different!

So how did she get it—this Girl Power? Did it show up wrapped in a nice, neat package on her sixteenth birthday? Was it magically revealed to her in a fantastic dream? Did her fairy godmother wave a magic wand and Girl Power descended in a cloud of pixie dust? Nope. None of the above.

The cool thing about Girl Power is that it's in *every* girl. That includes you, me and the girl sitting next to you in science class! **But you've got to discover it, respect it and *grow* it.** When you see a girl with strong Girl Power, you can bet that she's been growing it since she was a preteen. You can do the same thing, and there is no better time to start than now!

Let's Get Started!

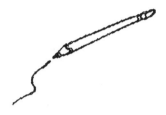

Girlology is about finding that special Girl Power and showing you how to let it do its thing. First you will need three sharpened #2 pencils, two clean erasers, 10 pieces of wide-ruled notebook paper . . . just kidding! *Girlology* is *nothing* like a school assignment or a test. It's meant to be read at your own pace. **Pondering is encouraged!**

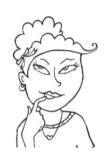

Remember we told you that there are some things that will just happen *to you* because you're a girl, and other girl things you have *choices* about? Well, we girls are going to talk about both in this book. We are going to challenge you to make decisions now about what choices you will make in the future. When you decide what is important today, you can make promises to yourself that you can stick to as you get older. These promises you make to yourself are important promises to keep!

We Need to **Talk**

When it comes to sexual things, you are going to want to talk about them. **And *everyone* is going to be telling you *something* about sex.** Here's where your Girl Power comes in—it's up to you to decide who can be trusted with your thoughts and feelings and who you can trust to give you good information. You will find out that some people want to tell you things about sex for your good, and other people want to tell you things about sex for their good.

All right, let's start with the "for your good" crowd. These are usually people like your parents, your family, doctors, nurses, religious leaders and teachers. Close friends can also be great, especially when it comes to sharing your thoughts and feelings, but they may not know all the facts about sexual things.

As for the "for *their* good" crowd, these people want to sell you stuff, persuade you to do what makes *them* feel good or show off. They are usually advertisers on TV and in magazines, certain movies and TV shows, and some friends or boyfriends.

The trick is to listen to people who can help you decide what is important to you and good for you—people who can help you decide on values you can stick to for the rest of your life.

How you think and feel about yourself, your body, sex and sexual things are important stuff. **You need to ask questions and get real answers.** You need to share your feelings and know they will be kept private. And you can only do this with someone you trust. *Girlology* will help you decide who is worthy of your trust.

But It's Kind of **Embarrassing**

Lots of things you read in this book will be good things to bring up with your mom, your dad or another trusted adult. Think those adults

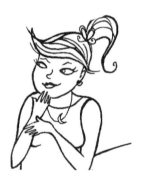

are clueless? Hopeless? Completely and utterly out of touch? Well, you'll be surprised to know that they were not dropped on this planet as adults. They actually had to go through the same stages that you are going through to become sexually mature. And while that may have happened in the "dark ages," most of them really do remember a lot about it.

Think your parents will be embarrassed by sex talk? They might be. *You* might be. But we promise that the more you talk about it, the easier it will get—for you *and* for them.

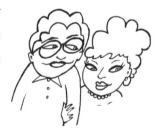

Puberty

We don't really talk about puberty a lot in this book because most of you are already in the midst of it or well beyond the beginning stages. Just to give you a definition, *puberty* is the time during a girl's or guy's life when they are becoming more adult- like in their body, including their appearance and their thinking. The word *puberty* comes from two different Latin words. One is *pubertas,* which means "adult-like," and the other is *pubescere,* which means "to grow hairy or mossy." Nice. Puberty starts for girls between the ages of eight and twelve. The usual start is with breast development, although plenty of girls start with pubic hair instead. For guys, puberty starts a little later, around the ages of ten to fourteen. Their start isn't as obvious because the first sign for them is that their testicles grow. Later signs for them are penis growth, facial hair and voice changes. Puberty lasts longer for guys than for girls. In fact, most girls are finished growing within two years after start- ing their periods. Guys sometimes don't finish growing until they are older teens, around seventeen to nineteen.

It's a **Life** Lesson

 Sex, breasts, periods, guys, body parts, Girl Power, choices, values, talking to adults—whew! That's a lot to learn, but we're going to make it interesting and fun. **It might occasionally be weird, too.** But hey, sometimes that can be the *most* interesting part!

Life lessons are supposed to be learned slowly. And that's what *Girlology* is—a life lesson. Remember, we're going to *grow* us some Girl Power . . . and growing takes time. So there's no need to race through this book. Read a chapter; think about it. Read some more. Think some more. Read. Think. Read. Think. Get the hang of it?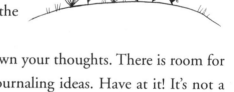

You might even want to write down your thoughts. There is room for that. There are some quizzes and journaling ideas. Have at it! It's not a school assignment, so have some fun. No pressure or grades!

The whole idea of a sex book may be freaking you out a little bit right now. Sexual maturing and growing up is confusing to *everyone* when it happens. But you know what? **It's just life.** You can't hide from it or ignore it—in fact, your changing body and brain will *make* you see it and think about it, sometimes a lot.

Girlology wants to take the mystery out of it all. Don't think of this as just a "sex book." Keep thinking of it as a life lesson. And when you finish this lesson, you'll have a better idea about who you are and who you want to become. You'll also have a plan for your sexual and relationship choices—a real plan using true information and based on your own values. A plan you can live with for years to come.

We know that girls are smart enough to make sense of all this confusing sex stuff. So turn on your brains, bring along your feelings and be prepared to discover great things about being a girl. Girl Power, here we come!

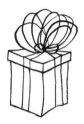

2

Friends Who Rock and Friends Who [Need to] Roll!

For most girls, **friends rock!** (Or do they?)

The middle school and high school social scene can be very strange—sometimes awesome, sometimes confusing and ugly. Girls say and do things to impress boys and other girls. Ditto for boys. Sometimes kids are nice to you; sometimes they're not. A trusted friend can suddenly be mean to you. Gossip abounds. There are cliques (pronounced "click"), clubs and groups that may embrace you or may make you feel left out. People you never knew before may suddenly seem more interesting than your old friends.

It may seem confusing now, but don't fear! There is a reason all of this is happening! Your brain is actually preprogrammed to help you accomplish two very important tasks before you become an adult:

1. Your brain is helping you to become more independent from your family.

2. Your brain is also helping you develop your values, your personality, your likes and your dislikes; you are figuring out who you are as an individual.

Now that's exciting stuff! Are you rolling your eyes right now and thinking that what we think is exciting is really too much grown-up stuff? Well . . . as a teen, you are sort of a "grown-up in the making." So bring those rolling eyeballs back to the page and read on!

Friends Over Family

Okay, so one of your jobs is to become more independent from your family. Believe it or not, your brain is programmed to make you want to

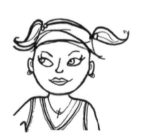

hang out with your friends more and your parents less. It's supposed to happen that way. You can tell your parents we said so.

Does that mean you abandon your family altogether? Nope. Does it mean you never hug, cuddle or play with your parents? Absolutely not! Does it mean that given a choice between going to the mall with your buds and playing a rousing game of Monopoly with your family, you pick your buds? Probably.

Things are going to change. It can be strange for you and your family.

Your parents are used to making all your decisions for you. They are used to having a little girl who looks to them for guidance and assurance. That doesn't totally stop, but now you are talking more to friends about important stuff, you are having your own ideas and you want more freedom to make your own decisions about where you go, what you wear and who your friends are.

Why Don't You **Trust** Me?

Raise your hand if you've ever said ". . . but why don't you trust me?" One, two, three, four . . . eight million, three hundred twenty-seven thousand, two hundred ninety-six hands . . . yep, your brains are working just fine on that independence thing!

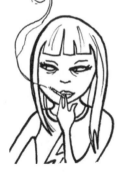

Independence is a very grown-up word. It doesn't mean "I get to do whatever I want to do, whenever I want to do it." Your brain tells you to become more independent so you can mature into an adult—not turn into a wild and reckless party animal!

The parents of all you party-animals-in-the-making also have a job to do as you gain independence. Their job is to make sure you can handle it. As much as it may bug you, your parents are doing their job when they want to meet your friends, give you curfews, supervise the clothes you wear and ask where you are going. That's what *their* brains are wired to do. We'll talk more about your parents in the next chapter. Let's get back to you and your independence.

Just in case you were getting a little nervous about the whole independence thing, relax. **You don't have to do it all by yourself.** Of course, you have your parents to help you along the way, but you also have friends. A group of friends is super important as you become more independent and figure out who you are. It can be kind of hard, though, because there are all kinds of cliques and groups, and you may not be sure where you fit in. Sometimes you feel more comfortable with your family; sometimes you click with one group of friends, sometimes with another group.

Time to figure out where you fit in!

Who Am I?

Huh? You don't already know who you are? Well, you have a name, an address and a birth date. That's a start. Take a look in the mirror. You have a unique look and a personal style.

Those are some of the givens. **But who you are depends more on the decisions you make, ways you act, stuff you experience and challenges you take on.**

"Who am I?" is a deep question. Thankfully, it doesn't have to be totally answered right now. Whether you know it or not, your brain is causing you to do things, have feelings and make choices that are getting

 you closer to the answer. It's a question you will be working on your entire life. But for now, you can't help but deal with it a little bit . . . and sometimes a lot.

Around your middle school and high school years, your brain sends you messages that you might not even notice. It's telling you to try new things, new thoughts and new ideas. This helps you "try on" some new things to see what fits. It helps you answer tough questions like: What's important to me? How do I want other people to see me? Is there

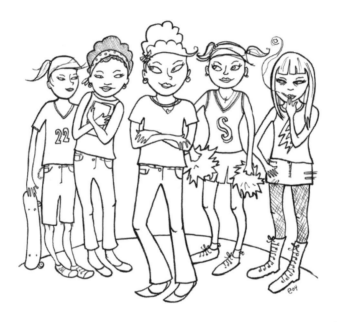

someone I look up to and want to be like one day? How will I dress? What will I look like, sound like, act like, be when I'm grown up? It's important to remember that you can't prevent these messages and impulses from your growing brain, *but* you can control the way you respond to them by staying in control of your actions and behaviors.

What are words you want people to use to describe you? Loyal? Fun? Intelligent? Clever? Creative? Patient? Kind? Artsy? Curious? Dramatic? Well, show them who you are!

For example, you decide that kindness is a trait that describes you.

Well, to be a kind person, you have to act like a kind person! (Surprise!) Begin noticing when you do and don't do things. Pick up a stranger's book when she drops it. Save a seat at lunch for your friend. Compliment a girlfriend on her new haircut. Fix your own lunch when your mom is running late. Find at least *one* nice thing to say about a girl that other girls are gossiping about. Want to be known as reliable and trustworthy? Then do what you say you will do. Keep the secret you said you would keep. Be on time. Call when you say you will call. Return the shirt you borrowed, and make sure it is clean!

People will know you by your actions. Actions really do speak louder than words. And it's all part of your brain telling you to be more independent. There are probably lots of qualities you want others to know you by. Maybe you see yourself as kind, creative and honest. Maybe you are generous, trustworthy and funny. How about creative, loyal and colorful? Pick a few qualities you'd like to show, and show them off! In many ways, you can choose what kind of person you want to be and then make it happen.

Words I want other people to use to describe me:

Things I can do so that people will see me as I want to be seen:

Friends—Are They Walkin' or Just Talkin'?

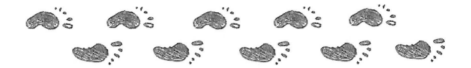

This whole "actions speak louder than words" thing helps you become the person you want to be . . . and it also lets you see what kind of people your friends really are. And when you know what other people are really like, that helps you know where you fit in.

Do you know any girls (or guys) who say they are your friends but then do things that aren't so friendly? Like the girl who spots you across the room in that new, cool jacket she saw at the mall and suddenly she is falling all over you, calling you "her new best friend" and asking you to sit at her lunch table? 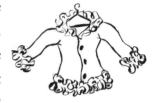 Then you find out she's telling other girls you think you're "so cool" because of your fancy new clothes? Seen it happen? Been there, done that?

Doesn't it make you angry? What that girl says and what she does just don't match up! That's called "talkin' the talk" (she says she is a friend) but not "walkin' the walk" (she doesn't act like a friend).

True friends encourage you and build you up. They listen. They focus on the good things about you. They are honest and loyal. They tell you when you have toilet paper stuck to your shoe or your shirt's on inside out. They say nice things about you to other people. They keep your secrets. They apologize when they mess up.

True friends *don't* tear you down, "dis" you or make you feel foolish. They don't gossip about you or focus on your weaknesses. They don't tell you that you look great when they know your fly is wide open or let you talk to your crush with broccoli in your braces. They definitely don't call you mean or embarrassing names, especially in front of other people.

Remember we talked about there being things that just happen to you (breasts, hips, pimples, periods) and other things you have choices about (when you kiss a guy, what you talk to your parents about, how you take care of your body)? Thankfully, friends are one of those things you get to choose!

And girl, you have some serious choices to make! We already know that your brain is telling you to be more independent, to spend more time away from your family and with your friends. The friends you choose to spend this extra time with are important! And the great news is that you have the power to make important choices like this that matter.

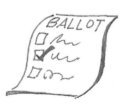 What do you value most in a friend? Trustworthiness? Loyalty? Rowdiness? Braininess? Humor? Religious devotion? Joyfulness? Truthfulness? Kindness? We could go on for pages and pages, because the truth of the matter is that you will choose friends with a combination of many traits you admire.

Try this. When you are deciding who will be in your close circle of friends, ask yourself: Is she walkin' or just talkin'? If her actions match her words, you have a friend worth keeping! Here are some examples:

Scenario	Talkin' the Talk	Walkin' the Walk
You have a crush on Luke. Luke asks your best friend to meet him at the movies. She knows that you would be hurt if you thought Luke liked her instead.	Your friend tells you that Luke is a loser so you won't like him anymore, and she meets him at the movie in secret.	Your friend tells Luke that she is flattered, but she can't go. She suggests that he calls you because she knows you don't have anything planned for Friday night.
The big party of the year is coming up. Your best bud is invited, but you aren't. One of the girls having the party tells your friend that she thinks you are a nerd and encourages her to come hang with the "popular" kids.	Your best bud tells you she has family plans, but she goes to the party anyway.	Your friend thanks the hostess for the invitation, but she hangs with you instead. She realizes that if they don't respect you for who you are, then they are not the type of people she wants to hang with anyway.

Scenario	Talkin' the Talk	Walkin' the Walk
Your friend is walking down the hall and sees you coming out of the bathroom. The hem of your cute skirt is accidentally tucked in your underwear, and your butt is almost showing. She's a long way down the hall.	She laughs hysterically, ducks into her next class and tells everyone about it.	She runs down the hall and quietly stands behind you, tells you and makes sure you get your skirt right.
You tell your best friend two big secrets. One, your parents are separating. Two, you are seeing a therapist to help you with your emotions. It's obvious you are very sensitive about these two issues.	Your friend acts all sad for you, but then you find out she told another girl that you are seeing a therapist so you must be "crazy."	Your friend offers emotional support and keeps your secrets. She is there for you whenever you need her, and she's a great listener.

Introducing . . . Miss Popularity!

Remember Girl Power? It's the confidence that lets you make choices that are good for you, even if they aren't the same choices everybody else is making. Well, get ready to use your Girl Power, because the crazy thing is that sometimes the most popular girls are the ones who tear you down and don't build you up. Go figure!

That kind of popularity is usually based on negative things. Some girls bully their way into being popular by intimidating or threatening people. Maybe they make you wish you had their gorgeous hair, killer clothes or good body. Maybe they flaunt their "sexiness" or put other people down. Lots of people seem almost afraid of this kind of popular girl because they don't want to be on her "bad side."

Oh, the glitz . . . the glamour . . . the fame of basking in the glow of the ever-popular, ever-beautiful, ever-manipulative girls! Yuck! **The bottom line is that choosing positive, caring, trustworthy friends might mean that you have to distance yourself from a particular popular crowd.**

That's the yuck side of popularity. But "popularity" is not always a word you choke down like a bitter pill. There are marvelous reasons to be popular. They are all reasons about who you are, what your strengths are, what your talents are and things you have in common with other people. All positive things about you!

Popular just means that certain people like you. The soccer goalie is popular with the athletic crowd. The guy who plays Romeo in the school play is popular with the drama crowd. The girl who reads to sick children at the hospital is popular with the community service crowd. Everybody can be popular in her own way!

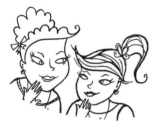

And remember that being popular is not the same as having a lot of friends. True friends know each other well, not just superficially. Just because a lot of people may know someone or may like her doesn't necessarily mean they are all her good friends. Consider yourself lucky if you have even one close friend who is the true, heart-to-heart, soul-to-soul, secret-sharing, help-you-through-anything, stand-up-for-you-always kind of friend. Now, *that's* more important than popular will ever be!

En Garde! Words as **Weapons**

Think about the last five times you got into an argument with a friend. What happened most often? Did you get your feelings hurt by something she said, or did she bust your lip with a vicious punch to the chin? We're betting your friend's weapon of choice was her words and not her fist.

The weapon of choice among girls—words?!? Well, think about it. **Feelings are fragile things, and some words can be like a sword piercing right through your gut!** Consider the following verbal attacks:

You help a guy friend with math homework, and another girl tells everybody, "She is so in love with him!" Ouch!

"Those jeans are totally Kmart." Ouch!

"Idiot!" Double ouch!

When you hear these things, think "Girl Power!" Am I an idiot? No. Am I totally in love with every guy friend I help out? No. Are my jeans Kmart? Well, maybe, but they are the cutest pair in town, so who cares?

Unfortunately, we can't control physical brain changes and hormones, so gossiping, insults, backstabbing and discouragement will always be around. **But remember, just because someone says it about you doesn't make it true.**

Of course, piercing words aren't just what "other girls" use. Your brain is telling *you* to fit in; it's telling *you* to join a group separate from your family; it's even telling *you* to exclude people from your circle of friends. Hey, brain, cut that out!

What Kind of Friend **Are You**?

Whew! That's a pretty unpleasant picture we've painted. So are middle school and high school nothing but a bunch of mean girls tearing each other to pieces? Heck, no!

While you can't control the physical things that happen to you, you can control (Girl Power!) how you react to them. Once again, we get to balance the things we can't control (brain and hormone changes) with things we can control (actions). We can choose to put down that sword, retract those claws and be a good friend to those around us. The Golden Rule is the perfect guide for friendship: **Treat others the way you want them to treat you.**

Remember that all middle and high school girls' brains are giving them signals to be more independent and try on new ideas, actions and attitudes. You don't need to totally drop a friend the first time she is mean to you. People change! Maybe that same girl just tried on a "snobby" personality for a couple days and found it didn't fit. Remember, you're all working through this together.

A great way to *have* true friends is to *be* a true friend. Remember that you will be insulting and you will gossip about other people. Some girls will do it more than others, but a good friend will apologize (and mean it) when she messes up. And good friends accept apologies graciously.

Now we get to the meat of friendship . . . what kind of friend are you? Do *your* actions match up to your words? Do you treat other people the way *you* want to be treated? When you choose friends by asking yourself, "Are they walkin' or just talkin'?" ask the same about yourself. Remember that list of words you want other people to use to describe you? **Do your actions make those things true about you, or is it just talk?**

What have you done lately that was "just talkin'"?

1.

2.

3.

What have you done lately that was really "walkin'"?

1.

2.

3.

Cliques

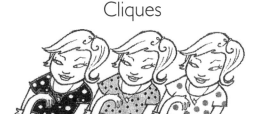

What do you look for in a friend? Does a girl have to wear the trendiest clothes? Be athletic? Read two novels a week? Wear black all the time? Play in the band? Be a drama queen, a cheerleader or a yearbook staffer?

You've seen the groups. They hang out together, eat lunch together, and sometimes even dress and act alike. Lots of groups have names. In most schools there are jocks, cheerleaders, preppies, goths, brainiacs, druggies, gearheads and artsy-fartsies. Your school probably has other groups that don't have such stereotypical names but are just as well-known. Can you name them?

Preteen and teen girls have a funny way of defining their groups. Clique is one way to describe a group of people who hang together. The word *clique* is usually used in a sort of negative way. Cliques can give "outsiders" a negative feeling because a lot of cliques don't let anyone else in, and they can be snobby and mean about it.

Have you ever seen a group make fun of other people who aren't like them? **When groups of people get together, they feel a lot more powerful than any one person would ever feel alone.** In a group, people will do things they would never do on their own—sometimes mean things or risky things. At the head of many cliques is a leader who likes control. Some of these leaders win friends by insisting on loyalty and making people scared they will be excluded if they don't go along with everything the leader says.

But there are also good leaders. They are the girls who gather people leaders win friends by insisting on loyalty and making people scared they will be excluded if they don't go along with everything the leader says.

But there are also good leaders. They are the girls who gather people together based on shared interests. They welcome new friends into the group. And they allow you to have other friends outside of the group. They don't boss their friends. These types of groups also have more power than any one individual would have, and they can accomplish powerful and amazing things—good things.

You may even belong to several different groups. You can be a soccer player and a braniac at the same time. You can share common interests with your neighborhood friends and your friends from your religion's youth group. The girls you meet at a Red Cross babysitting class can even become a clique because you all share the same job.

You may be in a group or clique yourself. Do other people have a special name for your group?

Who is in your group?

What do all the girls in your group have in common?

Do you welcome other girls or exclude them?

Outsiders and Feelings of **Isolation**

We hate to keep bringing up the yuck side of cliques, girl relationships and brain changes, but these things are important. **Feelings of isolation and being on the outside are normal and real.** *Really* real. At some point, almost everyone experiences these feelings a little or a lot. They happen to you and every one of your classmates.

For starters, kids who make other people feel isolated and on the outside on purpose are not worth a minute of your time. That just had to be said. We know that's an easy statement to make and a tough statement to live by. But we also know that it is true!

Girls who want to make other girls feel left out use some pretty sneaky tactics. They'll tell secrets, start rumors, exclude you, give you the silent treatment or manipulate you with confusing talk and demands. They may try to "steal" your other friends by monopolizing their time or telling them bad things about you.

They may also use more obvious tactics like putting you down and making snide remarks in front of other people. They may tease you, harass you and reveal secrets you told them. They may even attack you physically. And sometimes they can totally ignore you and exclude you, like you are invisible or a puff of smoke they brush aside with a wave of the hand.

Feeling ignored, unknown and invisible can be the worst feeling of all. If it happens to you, you can believe it has happened to a lot of other girls, too. When you find someone who has had the same feeling, it's almost a relief to know you are not alone, and better yet, you are not invisible! Nobody is. **Sometimes it just takes finding the friend who sees you well.** People who ignore you are just looking at superficial stuff. They obviously don't know who you are on the inside—the real you.

We'll let you in on a big secret. People put other people down to make themselves feel better . . . that means the popular girl who makes a snide comment about a classmate may be a little jealous. She probably sees something in another girl that she doesn't have. That kind of bully wants to make her "prey" feel bad about themselves, so the bully can feel like she has power over them.

So how do you handle it? What does a bully hope to get by bullying? Power. **How do you keep the power away from a bully?** You don't give her what she wants, which is usually crying, feeling bad about yourself and sucking up to the bully. *You have control over how you respond.* You don't have to feel bad about yourself just because someone wants you to. And you know what's really cool? If the bully doesn't get any power from you, she will leave you alone.

Boy . . . Friends?

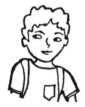

Now through this whole thing, we have mostly talked about your girl-friends as being your best friends, but we need to back it up a minute. What about friends who are boys?

Before we go any further, let's set the record straight so we don't get confused. When we talk about your friends who are boys, we mean boys that you don't have a crush on and don't have romantic interests in . . . we'll call them guy friends. When we talk about the boy you hang out with and have romantic feelings for, a special boy you like and who likes you back . . . we'll call them *boyfriends*.

And then there are guys you have a crush on, but they don't necessarily like you back in that same way. Your crush could be a famous singer who's never met you or a guy in your math class who doesn't even know you. Maybe it's the boy next door who thinks of you as a little kid or the lifeguard you met this summer at the pool. Anyway, it's a person who gives you "happy" butterflies in your stomach and someone you like to think about being romantic with, someone you want to know more about and someone you might think about a lot. We'll call them *crushes*.

It can get pretty confusing because your crush can become your boyfriend and a boyfriend should definitely be a crush. A guy friend can become a boyfriend or a crush and vice versa. So you see, **all these friendships can overlap and get all tangled up to the point that you're not really sure how to define the relationship.** That's okay, too. Nobody is going to give you a test on it. It's just the lingo we'll use in this book to try to keep us talking the same language.

Lots of girls have great guy friends. Sometimes it's easier to talk with a guy friend than it is to talk with your girlfriends. Guys and girls have different points of view on the same question. Guys and girls think differently, too. Something a girl thinks is a huge deal may be hardly worth talking about for a guy, and vice versa. Your guy friends can help you understand the ways boys think ("Boys think?" you say? Contrary to popular belief, they do!) and help put some things in perspective for you. Both girlfriends and guy friends are valuable friends.

Nothing More Than **Feelings**

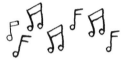

There's a fairly goofy old-school song that goes, "Feelings . . . nothing more than feelings. . . ." *Nothing more* than feelings? Ha! It's more like nothing more *important* than feelings!

Feelings will affect your friendships, your relationship with your parents, your interactions with teachers and your response to your siblings all day every day—especially while your brain is sending you those "Who am I?" messages. **The tough thing about feelings is that they can grab hold of you with lightning speed** even when it's not a reasonable feeling based on truth. Based on truth? Here's what that looks like:

 A girl at school calls you a loser. Are you a loser? No, but you still feel insecure.

 You get a bad grade on a test. Was the test unfair? No, but you still feel angry at your teacher.

 A classmate makes fun of the car your mother drives. Is a minivan a perfectly good mode of transportation? Yes, but you still feel defensive.

Feelings aren't bad, but the way we express feelings can be bad. **Check your feelings against the truth of what's happening.** That first feeling that sweeps over you may change!

Agree to Disagree

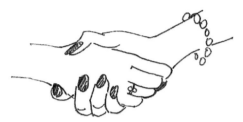

Tolerance. It's a word that gets tossed around a lot these days. Everyone has a right to her opinion, her own likes and dislikes, and her own ideas. **Being tolerant of other people's opinions doesn't necessarily mean you agree with them.** Tolerance means you put up with things (opinions, beliefs, actions, appearances) that you may not agree with. It doesn't mean that you don't have opinions of your own or that you can't argue your own opinion. It simply means you have to listen to the other side, be open to new ideas and agree to disagree if you don't find common ground. Learning to agree to disagree is part of learning tolerance and respect.

Tolerance also means that people can behave, dress, speak and look different from you, but you learn to accept them for who they are, even if you don't like what you see or hear (as long as they are not physically or emotionally hurting you).

All of our differences make up the diversity in the world. Tolerance is accepting the diversity and learning to appreciate it for making the world an interesting place. You've probably heard it before, but it's worth saying again . . . if everyone in the world were the same, the world would be a very boring place! **We are good at enjoying the things we have in common with our friends, but we have to learn to respect and appreciate our differences as well as our similarities.**

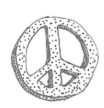

You can respect someone's opinion without agreeing with it. Learning respect and tolerance can be tough, but it's important. It helps you keep the peace with people who are different from you. That's how we can each contribute to peace on a larger scale—in our schools, in our cities, in our countries, even in the world. Not to be corny, but there's a great song about it: "Let there be peace on earth, and let it begin with me. . . ." It's about tolerance and respect. These are good things to remember when you are building your Girl Power.

What Do You Do with Feelings?

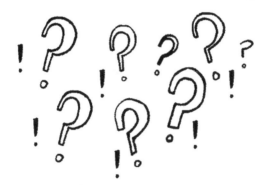

Feelings are a big-time part of friendships. Friends can make us feel happy, comfortable, content and safe. But some friends can give us bad feelings by making us feel jealous, embarrassed, threatened or angry.

What do you do when you have these bad feelings? Do you explode in a fit of angry words? Do you punch something? Or somebody? Do you hold it all inside and erupt like a volcano later on? Do you cry? Put yourself down? Hang your head in shame?

No doubt about it, feelings have to be expressed. Having feelings is *not* one of those things you have a choice about; **how you respond is a powerful thing you can choose.**

Okay, let's start with the punching response. Smacking someone across the face will always make the situation worse. Once the punching starts, everyone totally forgets what they are arguing over. Lots of black eyes, bloody noses and scratch marks. No solutions.

Instead, try sentences like these:

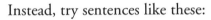 I don't like it when you drive too fast because it makes me feel scared.

I don't want you to touch me like that because it's uncomfortable for me.

I don't agree that she's a nerd just because she likes classical music.

That's not true. You can get pregnant the first time you have sex; I read it in our health book.

It's not fair to exclude her just because she wears black fingernail polish.

Use words! State your case! It will help you release your feelings even if the other person just argues back.

But what if that doesn't really work? What if you still are boiling with emotion? First of all, if anyone hits you, bullies you over and over again or makes you feel ashamed because they talk dirty to you or touch your body in ways that make you uncomfortable, go to an adult for help!

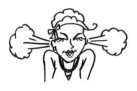

None of these things should happen to you. You deserve to be protected from this kind of bullying and abuse, and the people who do it should be stopped!

That's the worst-case scenario. But usually your feelings overflow from a personal disagreement. Step back, get away from the situation that has you all wound up and cool down. Count to ten. Grab a piece of paper, and write down your feelings. Write a letter to yourself, a letter to the person who caused your feelings to erupt or a journal entry. Talk to someone about it. Send the letter if you want, or rip it to shreds if that feels better. **Get it out and let it go, or get it out and *do something* to help the situation!** A lot of times, just getting your feelings out with your voice or on paper can help a ton!

Need **Help**?

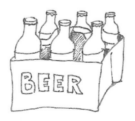

Sometimes the pain of feelings can get so bad that you may be tempted to "deaden the pain." That's when some girls and guys turn to alcohol and drugs to get "high" and "forget about it." They may look for sex to feel wanted. Some may try self-mutilation (scratching, cutting or hurting yourself in other ways) to block out bad feelings with physical pain or to get rid of "numb" feelings.

What? Are you crazy? Cut myself just because I'm angry? We know that's what some of you are thinking. But some of you may have already tried it, thought about it or know someone who has done it. It's a painful, desperate situation and more common than we'd like to think. It can be a cry for help when you don't know exactly how to get help. And if your friends are encouraging you to use sex, drugs, alcohol or cutting to "feel better," they need help, too.

Find someone you trust. If not your parents, maybe a teacher, a coach, a religious leader or another adult relative. Believe it or not, they went through the exact same changes you are going through. They might be surprised, but they may have had some of the same thoughts and fought similar battles. They have most likely known someone or even helped someone dealing with the same stuff. And they can help you get the kind of help you need.

If you're afraid to talk to an adult, ask a friend to find help for you. If you know of someone doing these things, tell an adult. Sex, drugs, alcohol and cutting are not secrets you want to keep. In fact, they are dangerous secrets to keep.

How do you know when you are getting angry?

How do you express your anger?

How can you deal with your anger better?

So, What's the **Point?**

So why did we have to go through the good, the bad and the ugly on friendships? **The point is that everyone your age is going through the same thing.** Everyone is trying to accomplish the normal and necessary task of growing up—becoming more independent from their families and figuring out who they are.

That means that there are a lot of confused and mixed-up kids roaming the halls of your school and the streets of your neighborhood. Guys and girls are growing into new bodies, changing friends, trying new things, experiencing unusual emotions, expressing themselves in interesting ways and figuring out their own feelings. Plus they are trying to figure out why everyone else is acting the way they are!

Whew! That's a lot to do. But it explains why your best friend turns mean one day and is back to normal three days later. It explains why the boy you've known since preschool, the same one you played cops and robbers with in first grade and soccer with in third grade, suddenly looks "cute" to you in sixth grade. It explains why you want to crawl into your dad's lap one day and then think he is an embarrassing dork the next.

It can be strange, but it *definitely* is normal. You are trying on new personalities, new friendships, new ways of thinking and figuring out where you fit in. One of the hardest parts of growing Girl Power involves learning how to be and how to find good girlfriends (and guy friends). **You can't control what your friends do or who they become, but you have the power to choose friends who bring out the best in you.** So let the bad friends roll, and you rock on, girl *friend*!

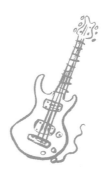

3

Where Have All the Normal Parents Gone?

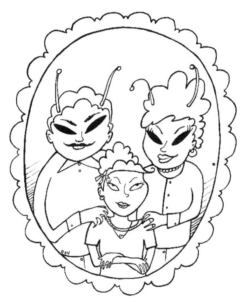

So one night your parents go to bed normal, nice, reasonable people, and the next morning they wake up **random, clueless, goofy aliens**. Sound familiar?

But wait a minute. Before we talk about how weird parents can seem to teenagers, let's talk about parents in general. While the traditional family with a mom, a dad, some kids and a few pets is still strong, there are lots of other types of "parental arrangements." Some kids are raised by a stepparent, some by a grandparent, some by only a mom and some by only a dad. Some are raised by a guardian, some by a parent and his or her "partner," and some by other parent substitutes. Other kids have one parent for a few days a week and another parent for the other days. That means some kids are dealing with four "parent types" on a regular basis!

The possibilities for parental arrangements seem endless, but do you get the picture? Parents come in all shapes, sizes and colors. They can be wrinkled grandmas, necktie-wearing salespeople or entrepreneurs with an office in the basement. They can be blood relatives, adoptive parents, family members by marriage or foster parents.

So when we talk about parents, we want you to envision the adults in your life who sign your permission slips. They are the people who buy you food, clothing, shelter and the occasional movie ticket. They discipline you, love you and protect you. If you don't have the traditional family of mom, dad, brother, sister, Fido . . . you are definitely not alone, and all this parent talk still applies to you. When we say "parents" or "mom" or "dad," you can read that however it fits in your life.

And now back to the topic we've all been waiting for—clueless parents!

Ch-Ch-**Changes**

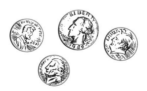

Okay, we know that preteen and teenager brains and bodies are changing. But what about parents? Do they seem to be morphing into more nagging, embarrassing, uninformed beings every day? Is it them? Is it you? Let's settle this issue fair and square . . . quiz time! Check "T" or "F."

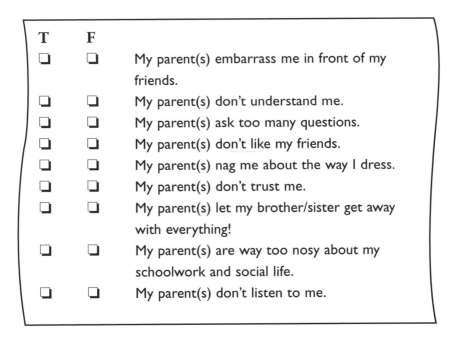

T	F	
❏	❏	My parent(s) embarrass me in front of my friends.
❏	❏	My parent(s) don't understand me.
❏	❏	My parent(s) ask too many questions.
❏	❏	My parent(s) don't like my friends.
❏	❏	My parent(s) nag me about the way I dress.
❏	❏	My parent(s) don't trust me.
❏	❏	My parent(s) let my brother/sister get away with everything!
❏	❏	My parent(s) are way too nosy about my schoolwork and social life.
❏	❏	My parent(s) don't listen to me.

If you answered true to any of these questions, guess what? You're normal. You're like a lot of teens, in fact, a vast majority of teens, who think their parents "just don't get" them. Why are parents that way? This may come as a big surprise, but it's a little bit about them *and* a lot about you.

The funny thing is that your parents probably haven't changed the way they are; they are just dealing with teenage issues now. These issues are different and more serious than little kid things, so parents may seem more strict and annoying in the way they guide you.

The real difference is the way *you* see them and respond to them. Your perception of your parents is changing pretty quickly!

But **Why?**

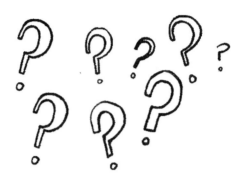

Remember how your body is changing, and your brain is changing, too? Those brain changes make you see your parents a little differently. When you were younger, you expected your parents to be totally involved and physically present in every aspect of your life. You may not have liked the *rules,* but you liked your parents *being there* because you needed their help. The world was bigger and scarier, and you relied on your parents to guide you through unfamiliar situations.

Well, now that you've been around longer, the world is not such a scary place. You can walk to a friend's house without getting lost. You can heat up pizza in the microwave. You can stay at home by yourself without being afraid. You can check out library books, make phone calls, pay a cashier and even be in charge of younger children.

Now when your parents give you limits and rules, you don't think, "I feel safe." You think, "Hey! You're trampling on my independence!" And that's a normal response. The bottom line is that **you *and* your parents have to grow into your new independent being.** They will have to change their rules and their limits to allow you to be more independent. You will have to earn independence bit by bit.

Be patient! Most parents want what's best and safest for their kids. The more you prove that you can be responsible with the little things (chores, keeping up with your own stuff, calling when you get to a friend's house), the more independence they will give you. *Voilà!* Everyone is happy!

You **Grow**, Brain!

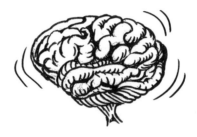

Just as your body has to grow into an adultlike body, your brain has to change into an adultlike brain (sound creepy?). And just as your body takes years to grow all those "woman parts," your brain takes your entire teen years to grow.

Two particular parts of your brain are growing like crazy! The first big grower is the part that helps you understand things like algebra. That's why we don't learn algebra in the second grade—our brains couldn't handle it! The same area in your brain also **lets you understand "invisible" things** like faith, trust, feelings and values. That's why you may be questioning the faith and values of your family. While it can be a little unsettling, kind of like thinking without a safety net, don't be afraid to question. Your parents may have taught you well, but your brain is now telling you to claim faith and values for *yourself.* Go for it!

Another brain part, your amygdala (uh MIG duh luh), is also cookin' away. This is the **emotional center** in your brain. By growing, it makes you experience emotions in a stronger way than you have before. You will begin to have intense feelings like anger, love and sadness.

While your amygdala is growing, it also interferes with your ability to figure out what emotions other people are feeling by their facial expressions, body language and tone of voice. So when you see a parent (or friend) with a wrinkled forehead and squinted eyes, you might jump to the conclusion that she is angry when in reality she is confused or worried or maybe just has a headache!

Your emotional center also makes you respond with big, lightning-quick emotions—like a firecracker popping. So that parent who was confused makes you suddenly explode with an angry yell before you realize that she wasn't angry at all. Then she *does* get angry because you yelled at her, and then your anger gets even bigger. Yada, yada, yada . . . **what a mess it can cause!**

See what we mean when we say this "clueless parent" phenomenon is a little bit about them and a lot about you? You may feel like your parents spontaneously turned more angry, more controlling, more nosy, more whatever overnight, but the way you interpret their responses is really what's changing. There goes that brain, doing a number on you again!

My **Brain** Made Me Do It!

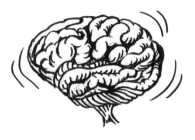

Besides these brain centers that are changing, scientists have also identified specific "developmental tasks" that you need to accomplish during your teen years. When you were a child, your "developmental tasks" were things like learning to sit, walk, talk, pick up a Cheerio with your finger and thumb, and potty train.

Now that you can successfully navigate a toilet (we're sooo impressed!), you get to move on to new tasks. Actually, they may seem more like annoying little chores. The most obvious tasks are physical ones like growing breasts, starting a period, getting taller, growing hips and growing new hair. Your major mental/emotional tasks aren't as obvious as breasts and pubic hair, but they still happen to everyone!

As we talked about, the first task is to become more independent from your parents and more connected with your friends. If you are ever going to become a responsible, independent adult, of course, **you have to learn to do things all by yourself.**

This parent-friend combo helps you accomplish your second big mental/emotional task—figuring out the deep question of "who you are." That means you consider your parents' values and your friends' values, and then you decide what's important to *you*. What kind of person do I want to be? What are my talents? What are my weaknesses? What will my family, my career, my faith and my accomplishments look like in ten or twenty years?

We talked a lot about this in chapter 2. If you're still wondering how to start figuring out "who you are," go back and check it out again.

Invasion of the **Body** Snatcher

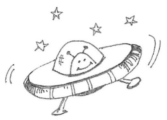

None of this is to say that your brain is holding your entire body, mind and personality hostage! When your brain gives you those "I need to be independent" messages, it may make you want to lash out with arguments, insults and disobedience when an adult challenges your independence.

Likewise, your brain may make you want to respond with anger, snide comments or unfriendly threats when your friends (or you!) try on "new" personalities on your quest to find out "who you are."

You can't control the messages your brain is sending you. Really. It's just the way your brain develops. **But you do have control over how you respond to your brain's messages.**

Right now you argue so much because your brain is also developing logical reasoning. You need reasons for your parents' rules; you want to know why your friends act the way they do. So ask your parents what purpose they have for a rule instead of responding with, "You can't make me!" Even if you don't like their reason, they probably have one that seems good to them. Once you know their purpose, you can negotiate a compromise that gives you some independence and also sets limits they think are good for you.

It works like this: Let's say you want to go see a movie, *Selena's Summer Secret* (a made-up title), with some girlfriends and some guy friends. You ask your mom, and she's says, "Absolutely not." You immediately assume that she doesn't trust your friends, thinks you pick lousy friends and maybe even hates your friends. And you tell her so! Yep, the perfect beginning to the perfect argument!

Or . . . you could tell her calmly that you really want to practice doing things on your own and ask her why she doesn't want you to go. (Note the word *calmly*. You are seeking information, not a fight here!) You choose this route and find out that it's not the *friends* she doesn't approve of, it's the *movie!* Turns out she read a review online and found out that it has really graphic sexual scenes and even shows naked breasts right there on the screen!

Wow! She really did have a good reason. You would have been mortified to be sitting right next to Derek when they showed naked breasts on the screen! So now that you know her reason, you can compromise. You can still go to movies; just pick a different one—preferably one without naked people prancing across the screen! You get to do something all on your own, and your mom gets to establish some safe boundaries for your independence.

See, once you understand what your developmental tasks are, it helps you explain to your parents why you want to do things "on your own." Tell your parents that you want to learn how to do things that will ultimately help you take care of yourself as an adult. We're betting you'll get lots of "maturity" points for that!

Where's the **Instruction** Manual?

So how do parents handle your changing brain and your new task of becoming independent?

Oh, that's easy. They'll just turn to page 26 of the *How to Raise Teenagers Instruction Manual* and refer to the easy-to-follow steps found there in the middle of the page. **What?!? You didn't come with a manual?** No instruction booklet? Well, this *does* complicate things. . . .

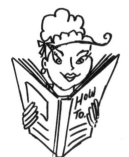

Looks like your parents are on their own when it comes to your changing brain and independent streak. Letting go of their little girl, deciding safe boundaries and giving up some control when it comes to safety, friends and your whereabouts isn't always easy. And it's different for everyone.

For some parents it's an easy task. For others it's torture. Some parents are happy that they don't have to watch you constantly anymore. Some might even give you more independence than you want. Lots of parents have already gone through this with older siblings and "know the ropes." Others are anxious first-timers. And some parents may never give up treating you like a six-year-old.

Parents with **Style**

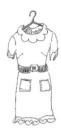

The way your parents handle these changes will depend a lot on their "parenting style." **"Style?" you say. "My parents have no style."** Ahh . . . you may be right, but we're not talking high fashion, clever conversation or cool cars. We're talking about the ways they discipline you, treat your friends and talk to you.

So what is your parents' parenting style? **Take this quiz,** and we'll help you figure it out.

✓ Check your parents' typical response:

Scene 1: A really cute guy invites you to a party at his house. You don't know him very well, but he hangs out with a bunch of popular boys who seem pretty nice. You ask your parents if you can go to the party with your best friend. Your parents respond with:

❑ *A. Wow, he sounds cute! Go get 'em, girl!*
❑ *B. You are not going, and that is final!*
❑ C. Who's having it? Where will it be? Will there be alcohol? Will there be chaperones? Who else will be there? What's his phone number so I can call to make sure his parents will be there?

Scene 2: Your best friend, who is usually very nice and innocent, comes over to go to the movies with you. She brings along some clothes for you to borrow, and you end up wearing her very short, very tight, very low-rise jean skirt and a shirt that is quite sheer. Your parents take one look at you and say:

❑ A. Hot outfit! Girl, you look good!
❑ *B. You are not going anywhere dressed like that.*
❑ C. I don't think your outfit is sending the right message to people about the type of girl that you are. If you are trying to look older, your red shirt and your own skirt might do a better job.

Scene 3: You and your boyfriend are going to a school football game. After the game, you want to invite him back to your house to hang out until his curfew. Your parents say . . .

❑ A. Great! We'll be out, but we'll leave the door open for you.
❑ *B. You spend too much time with that boy. Be home by 10:00, and we expect him to be gone by 10:15.*
❑ C. What time should we expect you? We'll be out, but we'll make sure to be home before you are.

Scene 4: Your friends are over jumping on your trampoline. You all start jammin' to some loud music, so loud that the neighbors complain. Your parents say:

❑ A. Kids will be kids. Nothing I can do about it.
❑ *B. Everybody inside! No more trampoline. You kids are too wild.*
❑ C. You are keeping the neighbor's kids awake with the loud music. How about turn the volume down to 5, and let's see if that helps.

The **Results**

$\mathcal{A}$ is for "**Always Cool**"

If you answered mostly $\mathcal{A}$, your parents may be acting more like a best friend than a parent. We'll call them Permissive parents. **Permissive** means that they let you do kind of whatever you want to do.

Woo hoo! Party time! Stay out late! Use Mom's credit card! Eat whatever I want! Hang wherever I want! Sounds like a blast, huh? **Your friends may think it's cool that your parents let you totally do your own thing, but teens actually do better and learn to have a healthier independence when there are rules.** That's not just what *we* say. Science proves it!

Permissive parents aren't necessarily trying to be "bad" parents; they just may be giving you **too much** freedom as you push for more independence. Kids who have a free-for-all with clothes, curfews and spending money often find themselves **wishing** for some guidance or someone who takes an interest in keeping them safe and on track.

Another way Permissive parenting happens is when your parents are acting more like a teenager than like a parent. They try to dress like you and talk like you. They might even hang with you and your buds and let you do adult stuff that a lot of parents wouldn't allow. Some parents think that they can take better care of you if they are your "best friend." **They mean well, but they don't realize that what you really need is a parent and not another "best friend."** If you have Permissive-type parents, we bet you know what we're talking about.

If you're in a family situation where there's not much supervision or interest in what you are doing or your parents are acting more like a teenager than you are, you can talk with another trusted adult like another relative, a friend's parent, a teacher, a coach or a counselor. They can help you establish healthy boundaries for yourself.

B is for "Because I Said So"

If you answered mostly B, your parents may want to make all your decisions for you. We'll call them **Authoritarian** parents. That means that they know what's right. Period. No discussion.

They truly may know what's right, but the problem is that **you can't learn to make good decisions if you don't know why your parents set certain rules.** If you don't have choices, even options they come up with for you to choose from, you end up with not much chance to prove yourself.

Use it or lose it. For certain parts of our brains, that's the way it works. Research shows that we have to start using the brain's decision-making center by adolescence. **If you don't learn to make some decisions for yourself, you will lose the ability to make good decisions later in life.** If someone else is always making decisions for you: what to wear, where to go, who to hang with, when to eat and sleep and do all the chores you have to do on a daily basis . . . you'll never figure out for yourself how to manage your time or your ability to decide things.

Authoritarian parents don't always mean to prevent you from ever learning to grow up, but they often don't give you the chance. So are they just control freaks? Maybe so, maybe not. It could be that you've messed up a lot and have given them a reason to think you can't make good decisions. Maybe you've broken lots of simple rules, so they think you can't handle bigger things. The best thing to do is promise them that you *can* make good decisions, that you *want* a *chance* to make good decisions.

Then do it! **Gain their trust—and trust is something that you have to earn.** Prove you deserve independence and then ask for more.

Sometimes Authoritarian parents may take their punishment too far. Sometimes they may be just too harsh and may even be abusive. If your parents leave marks on your body, lock you away or degrade you all the time, you've got a bigger problem than just "strict" parents. If any of that happens to you, it is important for you to tell someone you trust who can help you get out of danger. Sometimes your parents may just need some help learning better ways to discipline you, and sometimes they are just plain dangerous for you and your siblings. Kids who are abused by their parents can get help from people like school counselors, youth leaders, doctors, nurses or teachers. If it's happening to you, please talk to someone about it.

C is for **"Cooperators"**

If you answered mostly C, your parents are working hard to find a balance between your job of becoming independent and their job of giving you safe space to make your own decisions. We'll call them **Assertive-Democratic** parents. Assertive simply means that they state their case; they let you know what they think and why they think it. Democratic means that they often give you choices. It may not always be exactly what you want to do, but they will provide a number of safe options for you to choose from.

These parents know who your friends are, what your interests are, where you are and when you'll be home. **They are involved in your life but also give you room to grow some independence.**

Assertive-Democratic parents seem to provide the best opportunities for helping their kids make the transition into young adulthood. These parents don't just pop into this category, though. They learn by being Permissive sometimes, Authoritarian sometimes and then discovering the balance of Assertive-Democratic. Since you didn't come with an instruction manual, parenting involves a lot of trial and error!

Being a teen also involves a lot of trial and error. You have to discover which category your parents seem to hang out in. Maybe you have one parent who is Permissive about clothes and Authoritarian about schoolwork. Another is *usually* Assertive-Democratic about your social life but occasionally swings to Authoritarian when it comes to dating. Confusing? You betcha!

When you look at your parents, you'll probably see a combination of Permissive, Authoritarian and Assertive-Democratic qualities. That can be good. Even parents who are 100 percent Assertive-Democratic have good reason to be what you may think is Authoritarian or Permissive at times. They may need to tell you what to do absolutely, period, no discussion if it is an issue you have already discussed, involves a choice you have already been allowed to make, and you are making a poor choice for the third time.

They may seem Permissive if you are not taking responsibility for a decision they think you can make on your own. They may push you to decide between going to a friend's house and getting a jump-start on a huge research project if you have always counted on them to make that decision for you. In this case, their response, "Whatever you think is best," forces you to use your brain's decision-making center.

By now, we guess you are figuring out the truth about parents—they don't come with an instruction manual either!

How to **Get Your Way** with Your Parents

If you are going hog-wild with the independence thing by talking on the phone all night; eating nothing but pizza, mac 'n' cheese and soda; and buying a brand-new outfit every weekend . . . Hey, hey, hey! Slow down there!

If getting your way means unlimited phone calls, junk food and trips to the mall, you won't learn how to make that happen from us! We've already said that growing up does not mean that you get to do whatever you want to do whenever you want to do it. And getting your way with your parents isn't the same as having a rules-free home.

But if getting your way means "gaining independence," we can help you there! The real challenge is figuring out how to deal with these different parenting styles—Authoritarian, Permissive and Assertive-Democratic. You need a plan that allows you to gain independence and figure out who you are, but still lets your parents do their job of protecting you, loving you and raising you to adulthood.

The **Drill** Sergeant

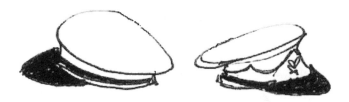

First, let's take a look at Authoritarian parents.

Authoritarian parents make clear rules which are unbending. They expect obedience, and breaking a rule is strictly punished. Now we're not saying that rules, boundaries and consequences are *bad*. In fact, they are really good for you. It's just that teens need some room to make decisions for themselves. And that can't happen if an Authoritarian drill sergeant of a parent directs every detail of your life with no explanation or choices.

For a healthy brain, a totally Authoritarian parenting style is not the best for teens. Remember use it or lose it? That decision-making center has to get some exercise, or you'll never be able to make decisions as an adult!

Even if your parents are not Authoritarian now, you probably remember a time when they were. Authoritarian rules work best for younger children, children who cannot fully understand the danger of running in the street, playing with fire or eating only chicken nuggets for three months. When you were a little older, your parents still may have had good reason to be Authoritarian. Maybe you wanted to see a movie that had sexual situations . . . but didn't even know what sex was yet! Your parents may have given you a reason for their rule, but you were too young to understand.

So at certain times in your life, unbending rules did have to be made *for* you, regardless of whether or not you understood the reasons.

That was then. This is now. **You are older and able to understand choices and consequences.**

Every time you make a decision, it's like exercising your brain. The more decisions you make, the more fit your brain's decision-making center will be. If your parents make all your decisions for you, that brain's gonna turn into a big tub of goo! Ewww!

So how do you get Authoritarian parents to "let you have your way" and make some decisions?

1. **Show them that you *do* understand that choices have consequences.** Use "I" statements, such as: "If you'll let me stay out until 10:00, I promise to be home on time. And if I'm late, I'll wash your car every Saturday for a month." And then if you are late, suffer your own consequences cheerfully.

2. **Do the small things well.** Make your bed without being reminded. Remember your lunch money. Finish your model of the solar system on time. Show them that you can do things on your own. Give them a reason to think that you will make good choices, and they may let you try bigger things.

3. **Tell them that you *want* to make some decisions.** Ask them to find times for you to exercise your brain. Make suggestions like: "Will you let me decide when I'll rake the lawn if I promise it will be done by Saturday at 6 P.M.?" or "Can I go shopping for that new skirt with my friends if I promise I won't buy one shorter than three inches above my knee?" or "May Amber and I walk around the neighborhood if we take the cell phone and promise to be back in thirty minutes?"

These things prove to your parents that you can set reasonable limits and accomplish tasks all on your own (home at 10:00, a school project finished on time, hem three inches above the knee). It can make them more confident that you *will* make good choices. They may even look pensively heavenward, lay a finger aside the cheek and ponder, "Maybe, just maybe, I don't have to make all my little girl's decisions. . . ." Your brain will thank them!

The **Sky's** the Limit

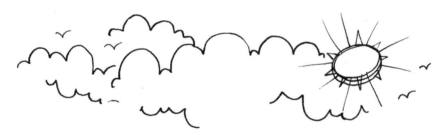

Now on to Permissive parents.

Permissive parents may be the toughest parents to deal with. We just saw how Authoritarian parents set up unbending rules about all details of life so that teens can't practice making decisions. Permissive parents are the opposite of that.

Permissive parents encourage kids to think for themselves, do whatever makes them feel good and avoid conformity. Misbehavior is usually ignored, and kids learn from making mistakes. Children of Permissive parents have lots of chances to make decisions—the sky's the limit!

It's just that teens need rules, limits and guidance to feel secure and *learn* to make good decisions. **If you don't have guidance about the**

pros, cons and consequences of making certain choices, it's gonna be tough for you to learn. You didn't drop onto this Earth as a completely developed 30-year-old "Ms. Responsibility." No! Your brain is *still growing* into an adult brain; you're not there yet.

It's sort of a role reversal to ask parents to give you more rules and limits, but really that's what's best for you and your developing brain. So how do you get Permissive parents to "let you have your way" *and* set some limits that help you gain good independence?

1. **Ask them for supervision.** For example, you could say, "I want to ask Joe over after the game to hang out, but I'm kind of uncomfortable being at home alone with him. Could you be home by 10:00?" Or maybe, "The neighbors just yelled across the fence that we are too loud. What can we do that's quiet but still fun?"

2. **Learn from your parents' actions.** They are making decisions every day, and you can learn from their choices and consequences. Maybe your mom turns down an invitation to go to a movie with a friend because she needs to help your little sister make a Native American Indian costume for school. You see the delight in your sister's eyes, and you know Mom made a good decision. Maybe your dad promises to be at your volleyball game, but at the last minute he decides to play golf after work with some buddies instead. You are disappointed and probably angry, and you know that was a bad decision.

   You can learn from good and bad choices people all around you make. Look to your friends. Read the newspaper. Check out what happens to characters in books, on television and in movies. Take note of consequences of your own actions.

3. **Look to other trusted adults for guidance and boundaries.** A friend's mom is a great choice. You'll know the right one when you meet her. She talks to you a lot, remembers things about you and explains her reason for choosing certain rules and boundaries for her daughter. She's fun in a "like to be around her" way, not a "party time, no rules" way. If you can't find a friend's mom to confide in, other good choices are teachers, coaches, religious leaders, neighbors or other relatives.

You may be thinking, "Sounds like fun! I want Permissive parents! Freedom, freedom, freedom!" Well, we know that giving yourself rules and limits seems totally bizarre. But remember that what you learn *now* forms the adult you will be. Decision making with guidance will snap that brain of yours into shape pronto—and you'll have the perfect brain to usher you into adulthood.

A Little **Me,** a Little **You**

And now for the crowning glory of teen parenting styles—Assertive-Democratic. Assertive-Democratic parents establish basic guidelines for their children. They give clear reasons for setting limits. They teach their children about the consequences of choices and give them plenty of practice making choices. If this is the type of parents you have, **you will be expected to take responsibility for the choices you make.**

While no parents are perfect, Assertive-Democratic parents seem to prepare their children best for being adults. Research shows that children raised this way make wiser choices, cope well with change and are better problem-solvers. In other words, they have strong, well-exercised decision-making centers in their brains. No tubs of brain-matter goo here!

Assertive-Democratic parents are already "letting you get your way" by encouraging you toward independence. But there are some things you can do to help out. It's a case of they give a little, you give a little.

1. **Learn from your mistakes.** Your parents aren't going to let you go jump off a cliff, but they will let you make relatively safe but poor choices. If you decide to IM your friends all night instead of studying for your geometry exam, you will discover the nasty consequence of failing. Prove to yourself and your parents that your brain gets just as much exercise from making bad decisions as it does from making good decisions—and decide to study next time!

2. **Ask their opinions about decisions you need to make.** While it's hard to imagine your mom having her first period, her first kiss and a curfew, we can assure you that she did. Just ask your grandma! Your parents have lived long enough to make many decisions— good and bad—and they can share their real-life experiences with you.

3. **Offer reasons of your own for making decisions.** This is when your parents will shout for joy, "Well, at least we did *something* right!" Making well-thought-out decisions is exactly what they have been training you to do. When they see that you have considered the consequences of a choice, they'll confidently grant you your independence. Yahoo! Mission accomplished!

So What Is **Normal**?

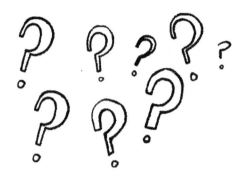

Let's review a laundry list of "normal" parent behaviors. They:

- Embarrass you
- Nose around in your business
- Fuss at you about schoolwork, clothes, computer time and your whereabouts
- Hate your friends
- Love your friends
- Establish strict, unbending rules
- Establish no rules at all
- Give you reasons for the rules
- Make decisions for you
- Let you choose

Yep, looks like all those abnormal, clueless parents out there are really pretty normal after all. Your normal parents didn't go anywhere . . . your relationship with them and your perception of them just changed.

Now that we know your parents are possibly and even probably normal, where do you go from here? That's easy. Keep heading the way your brain and body are leading you—straight toward independence. **No matter what your parents' parenting style is, that brain of yours will get its best exercise by making good decisions.** Do whatever it takes to get the best information you can to help you make the best decisions you can . . . and watch your independence grow! Your Girl Power will grow along with it!

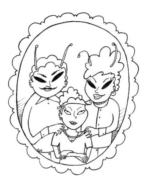

PART TWO

Body Talk

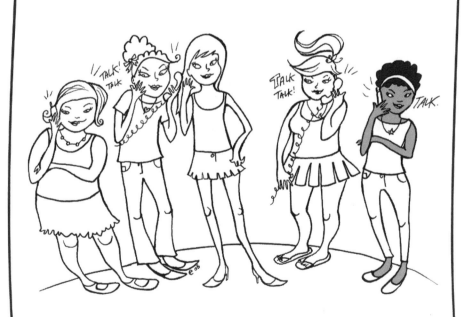

4

Not Your Usual Vocabulary List!

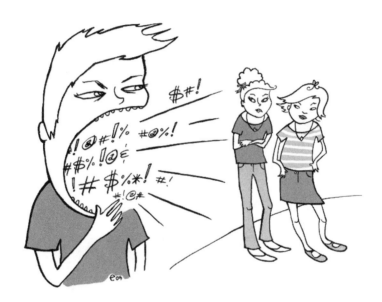

Words are powerful. You know because you use them all the time. You use words to get information when you ask your teacher, "Why did Shakespeare make men put on dresses, wigs and high heels to play women's roles?" You use words to stand up for yourself when you tell a girl in your class, "I'll help you with the math homework, but I'm not going to let you copy mine." And you definitely express anger with words when you scream at your sister, "You idiot! I told you not to wash my white sweater with your stupid red sweatshirt!"

When we're talking about our bodies and sex, using clear, accurate words gives us great power. Sex talk might be a little uncomfortable at first. There are lots of new words, and lots of words you'd only use with girlfriends—lots of words you'd never use with parents or teachers. Don't worry. In chapters 4 and 5, we're going to learn clear and accurate words for sex talk. And we're going to get you some more power!

Pop quiz! Define the following (25 points each): scrotum, clitoris, areola, coitus . . . just kidding. What? Never seen these in your English book? Just as we suspected . . . this will not be your usual vocabulary list!

Awkward Words

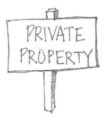

It's no secret that a lot of girls don't feel comfortable talking about their "private body parts" or things related to sex. It can be embarrassing. It can even be scary. A lot of adults don't feel comfortable talking about it either. It's normal to feel uncomfortable and awkward talking about sex and personal subjects. It's not something we go around talking to everyone about like the weather. But once you do start talking, it gets easier—for teens *and* for adults.

To help you understand some important things, you will need to know a lot of new terms and words. Some you know; some you don't know; some you say; some you don't say. There are also lots of words "out there" that you hear but may not understand. You need to learn about those, too.

Some of the words we think you need to know are listed below. Some words that we think you *don't* need to know are also listed below. We put them there because we know you hear them anyway, and you deserve to at least know what they mean, so you can find "better" words to use in their place. By the time you have finished this book, you should know what all of them mean. Beside the words we have listed, you can also add the slang words that mean the same thing (it's okay, really!). We want you to feel comfortable asking about words you don't fully understand. We also want you to feel free to add other words to this list. If we don't cover them here, ask a parent or another trusted adult. When you feel embarrassed, just remember that they probably feel just as awkward answering as you feel asking! Here's your new vocabulary list:

Abortion (termination of pregnancy)—An abortion is a medical or surgical procedure that removes a pregnancy from a woman's uterus to end the pregnancy.

Birth control (the pill, condoms, the patch, the shot)

Breasts (boobs, tits, titties, jugs, bosoms, bust)

Clitoris (clit)

Condom (glove, rubber, prophylactic, Trojan)

Douche—We don't know any slang terms for this one, but a douche is a device that some women use to wash out their vagina. It is not recommended. In fact, it can cause problems with infection.

Ejaculation (cum . . . see orgasm)

Homosexual (gay, queer, dyke, faggot/fag, lesbian, homo)

Horny (blue balls, hot)

Kissing (making out, sucking face, slipping the tongue)

Lust (crush)

Masturbation (jerk off, whack off, playing with yourself)

Menstruation (period, cycle, "aunt flo," monthly, the curse, my little friend)

Oral sex (cunnilingus, fellatio, going down, blow job)

Orgasm (cum/come, climax, the Big O)

Penis (dick, pecker, weenie, unit . . . and lots more!)

Petting (making out, feeling up, second base, third base, hand job)

Prostitute (whore, slut, skank)—A prostitute is a person who has sex for money, shelter, drugs or other "things."

Sex (sexual intercourse, coitus, making love, going all the way, doing it, doing the deed, getting laid, scoring, screwing, and yes, the f*** word)

Sexual harassment (coming on too strong)

Sexually transmitted infection (STD, clap, drip, herpes, crabs)

Testicles (balls, nuts, the family jewels, nads)

Uterus (womb)

Vagina (pussy)

"Bad" Words

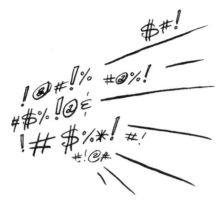

Did you read some words that flipped you out or made you laugh? Are you afraid that your mom is going to freak out if she reads this book now?

Sticks and stones can break my bones, but words will never hurt me. We know you've heard that old expression. It's true, kinda. Words won't really hurt you physically, but they can hurt your feelings and make you feel yucky about yourself.

And people use certain words that can make you, your body, your sexuality and sex seem nasty and cheap. Words themselves (even words about sex and your body) aren't bad. It's just that some people use words to put down what is the really beautiful, amazing and normal development of teenage bodies and sexuality.

Most of these "bad" words are about our body parts or things we do with our bodies. **Why do people feel like they have to use silly or not-so-nice words to talk about things that are a normal part of life?!** Can you think of some reasons people might do that? Maybe:

❑ They don't feel comfortable with the topic.

❑ They don't know the real or proper words to use for what they want to say.

❑ They are copying negative attitudes towards sex and bodies they see in movies, magazines, on the Internet and on TV.

❑ They think the words are funny or risqué to say, and they get attention by saying them.

Bet you can think of some of the words that people use when they could be using nicer, more proper words.

There's Nothing Wrong with a Little **Curiosity**

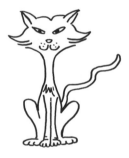

Trust us. Curiosity about words people use for sex and body parts will not harm you or get you in trouble. **It's how you use words that can get you in trouble.** In this book, there are no words that are "bad." There are just words you need to understand. Remember, curiosity is normal, knowledge is power and language is powerful! Just because you know what all these words mean doesn't mean you will start using them in your daily conversations (please!).

Understanding what different words mean helps you gain a little power over the people who use them in "not-so-nice" ways. When you hear people using "bad" words, you will know that they often do that to shock others, to be mean or to show off. Then you can look at them with a look that says:

"I think my body is pretty cool and amazing and beautiful,
and I'm not into talking nasty about it."

or

"Oh, you must be uninformed
since you don't feel comfortable using correct words"

or

"Oh, you must need extra attention . . .
don't you know there are better ways to get it?"

or

"Oh, that was mean, and I don't have time for mean people."

Get it?

The Look

By the way, preteen and teen girls are the best at giving "the look" we're talking about here. You know the look—rolling eyeballs, raised eyebrow (only one if you're really good), smug look and a quick, grunty sigh! It's okay to use it when necessary! It works (we bet you've already discovered that by now). Just don't use it too often because it will lose its effect.

The point is that when others use "bad" language, it doesn't make them stronger or respected or better than anyone else. It just makes them seem a little immature to those who have Girl Power. You can be bigger than that.

Hurtful Words

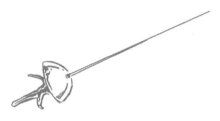

Some people will use "bad" language on purpose to make other people feel embarrassed or bad about themselves. That type of language insults others. Just because someone says it about you doesn't make it true!

Remember the "sticks and stones" thing? If someone uses "bad" language against you, don't let them feel they have won anything. Ignore them and be strong. Your feelings and your spirit might be hurt, but it's their character that is damaged. Remember that the people who use hurtful language are wimps, and you might even feel sorry for them (if you weren't so mad!).

It's Really Just a Big **Cover-Up**

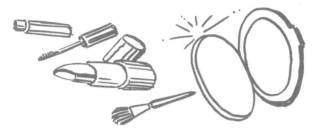

Most of the time, people who are mean like that don't feel very good about who they are, and one way they make themselves feel better is to bring other people down with them. So they say bad things to make others feel as bad as they feel about themselves. It's kind of sad, because **someone who feels good about herself would never need or want to put other people down.** A big part of Girl Power is feeling good about yourself, so you never need to act like that.

You also need to know about something called **sexual harassment.** That's when someone uses sexual language or talks about sex in a way that makes you feel uncomfortable, embarrassed or even threatened. It's another way that people use words or body language to try to feel powerful. The important thing to know about sexual harassment is that it is ILLEGAL. There are laws that protect people from being sexually harassed, especially in schools and in jobs. So if sexual words or actions are being used in this type of way, especially if it is happening over and over, it is very important to let a trusted adult know about it. Sexual harassment can be stopped!

What Does **That** Mean?

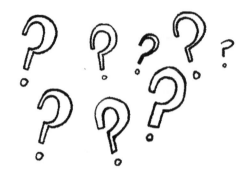

Another problem comes up when you don't know a word that you hear and you suspect it's one of those not-so-nice words. You get confused! It's hard to know whether someone just dissed you, insulted you or even sexually harassed you. If you come across a word like that, don't be afraid to ask what it means. If it isn't cool to ask the person who said it (because they might try to embarrass you), ask a parent or other trusted adult.

If you ask a parent, you should get an honest answer *and* some advice on how proper or improper the word is. *Don't* try to use the new word in a sentence to your parents to see how they react! Just tell your mom or dad that it came up in the locker room or hallway, and you were wondering what it means. Your parents shouldn't get mad at you for an innocent question like that. Besides, they should be happy that you are bringing your questions to them. If they freak out, give them a little time to cool down. **Parents get all flustered sometimes when they find out that you know stuff that they don't think you need to know.** Again, explain that you are just curious and didn't want to take your question to anyone else.

Almost all parents really want to talk to their kids about this kind of stuff, but most of them don't know how to start the conversations. This way, you've started it a little and opened the door for more talks in the future. **Sometimes, the kids have to lead the way!**

Words I might ask someone about if I get really brave:

Body Talk

What's with all the "cutesy" or slang words we use for body parts? You know them: my pee pee, my boobies, my titties, my coochie, my poopie, my butthole, my ass or "down there." **There are a gazillion silly sex-related words,** but why do we feel like we need to use them?

Comfort. 'Cause it can be downright awkward using the proper words, right? Can you say vagina without giggling? How about penis? Have you ever heard of a urethra? But we don't get all giggly when we say head, shoulders, knees and toes, so why do we get tickled when we talk about the parts "down there"? All those "parts" are just more parts of our body.

Let's say you get hit in the face with a softball and cut your upper lip on the inside of your mouth. Are you embarrassed to tell your doctor where you are hurt? What about if you slip while walking on a narrow brick wall, straddle the wall and cut yourself near the opening of your vagina? How are you going to explain where you are hurt?

There are lots of reasons why it's important to understand the proper terms for your anatomy. **It's your body. Get to know it!** The next chapter will take you on a trip "down there" to learn the words you need to know and to tell you what all those amazing parts can do!

5

Everybody's Got a Body

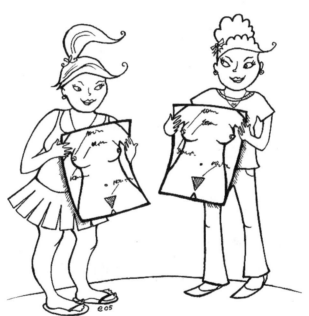

Tall, short, skinny, fat, muscular, sinewy, chubby, bean-pole. There are a million and one names that people use to describe bodies. Even though our bodies look different, they all have the same parts. Remember that what your body can do is more important than what it looks like. **All these amazing parts**

work together to let us do lots of awesome stuff.

When you were about two, you started learning the names for parts of your body. Your parents were so proud when you pointed your chubby little finger to your face and said "nose" and "eyes." They would brag to all their friends about how smart you were. Now, why on earth would they forget to tell you the names of your "private parts"? After all, when you were born, you can bet it was one of the first parts of you they wanted to see. Boy or girl? Girl! **Well yay, you are a girl.** So why not know the names for those girl parts? Even better, why not know what all those parts are for?!

When it comes to seeing what your private parts look like, we think boys have a major advantage. If you have ever seen a naked boy or man (we're thinking brothers, dads, little boys you baby-sit, but hopefully not someone running naked around your neighborhood), you probably noticed that their "private parts" aren't as private as girls' parts are. In fact, they are hanging and wiggling right there on the outside. When a little boy starts to potty train, he learns to hold his penis to aim it in the toilet . . . hopefully. So boys have been looking at and holding their private parts all of their lives.

For girls, on the other hand, we don't need to hold any of our parts to go to the bathroom (Look Ma! No hands!). And in case you've ever tried to look, you know we can't see much from above except some skin folds. Our private parts are a little more private, and they are pretty hard to see unless you use a mirror. You are probably crinkling up your nose and saying, "Ewwww, gross," right now. But there's nothing gross about your body parts. **Without them, you'd have some major problems!**

We encourage you to use a mirror to have a look. You might want to use a flashlight, too. Sometimes it helps to put one foot up on a chair or the toilet. Better yet, put your mirror on the floor and squat down over it.

Have you ever tried it? Are you grossed out? Don't be. Go
ahead! It'll probably feel a little awkward at first, but it's
painless, and actually pretty interesting. You look at your
face every day, right? You should definitely look at your girl
parts every once in a while, too.

For now, the main reason to look at yourself is **to sat-
isfy your curiosity and to get smarter about your body.** Once you
learn all the parts that girls have, you'll want to see for yourself that all
your parts are present and accounted for! At other times, like when you
use a tampon and later in life when you are involved in sexual activity,
there will be other good reasons to understand your anatomy and how
things work.

The easiest way to learn all the parts is to start with the "outside" parts
and then learn about the "inside" parts. The outside parts are what most
girls mean when they are talking about "down there." So let's go over
some of them.

The **Outside** Parts

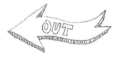

In general, the outside girl parts are called the vulva (not Volvo—that's
a car). It's a name that includes a lot of other parts, kind of like how your
face includes your cheeks, eyes, nose, mouth and so on. Your vulva
includes two holes, a lot of skin folds and some "padding." The definitions are listed below. You'll be expected to spell and use each word
correctly in a sentence at the end of this chapter . . . just kidding!

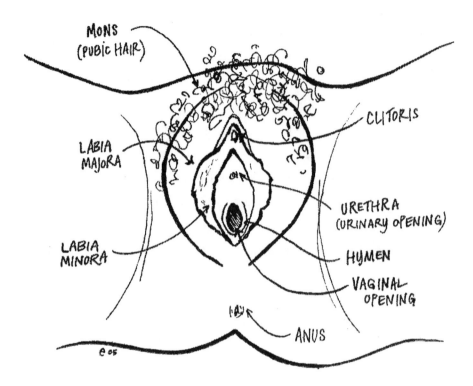

Vulva—the name for most of the outside "female parts," including the labia majora and minora, urethra, vaginal opening and the surrounding skin. It is also called "external genitalia." The word *genitals* refers to the body parts on boys and girls that are involved in making a baby (we'll get to that later). The parts of the vulva are listed next.

Labia majora—the outer lips that will become covered with hair as your body grows and develops. They provide a fatty layer of protection for the other sensitive parts of the vulva.

Labia minora—the inner lips. They come in lots of different sizes, shapes and colors, but for you, they should be about the same size on each side. They may be bigger than the outer lips. They may also look darker and wrinkled or they may be pink and smooth. Yours may not look exactly like the drawing, and that's okay.

Clitoris—the bump just inside the top of the labia. It contains tons of nerve fibers and is very sensitive to touch. Rubbing it or stroking it feels good and usually creates sexual pleasure for females. During sexual excitement, it may become a little bit bigger and stiffer. It is protected by a flap of skin called the clitoral hood. If you pull back on that skin, you can see the clitoris better (it won't hurt, go ahead and try it!).

Urethra—the "pee" hole or opening where urine comes out. It's the first opening below the clitoris. It is also pretty sensitive when touched or rubbed, but it's not a "feels good" kind of sensitivity. If the urethra is rubbed too much, it can actually become irritated and cause mild burning when you urinate.

Vaginal opening—the opening of the vagina (duh). It's not always "open," but it will open if you put something in it, like your finger or a tampon. More about the vagina when we get to the "inside" parts, too . . . bet you just can't wait!

Hymen—a small rim of tissue that is at the rim of the vaginal opening. It can be tender if you try to stretch it or push hard on it. Hymens come in a lot of different shapes and sizes, too. Once you reach puberty, the hymen becomes thicker and more elastic with a "ruffled" edge. That makes it kind of hard to see among all the folds and flaps "down there." Using a tampon will not necessarily tear your hymen because it can usually stretch to allow something that size through it. All girls are born with a hymen, but once you are a teenager, the way the hymen looks does not necessarily show whether or not you have had sex.

A lot of people put a big emphasis on the hymen because it supposedly "tears" and bleeds the first time you have sex. The reality is that some women or girls will have a small amount of bleeding when they first have intercourse, and some don't have any. It may just depend on how relaxed and ready for sex she is.

Perineum (pear uh NEE um)—the thicker tissue that is between the bottom of the vaginal opening and the anus.

Mons—the fatty mound where pubic hair grows in a shape like an upside-down triangle. The mons also provides a fatty padding to cover your pubic bone, which can hurt if it is bumped too hard.

Groin—the area on your front side where your legs are connected to your trunk. Pubic hair usually grows to this point or may grow past it onto your upper thighs. If you shave your pubic hair for your bathing suit line, you may notice some small "knots" in this area. Those knots are lymph nodes or glands that get bigger when there is irritation or infection on the skin (like razor rash or ingrown hairs). The knots should go away in time. If they become larger, tender or won't go away, see your doctor. You can help prevent razor rash and ingrown hairs by using soap or shaving cream and a new, clean razor every time you need to shave. Shave the hair in the same direction that it grows out of the skin.

Hair, **Where**?!

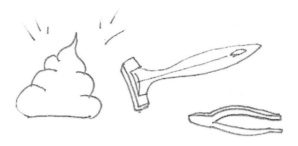

While we're on the subject of pubic hair . . . let's talk about whether to groom it or not. First of all, shaving or "de-hairing" legs and armpits is fine if you want to. Some girls don't. Some girls want to shave off all of their hair "down there." Is it a good idea? It's definitely okay to get rid of unwanted hair that might poke out of your bathing suit, but do you need to remove all of it? We think not. In fact, girls who remove all of their mons hair can develop skin infections that become big abscesses full of pus. Ewwww and ouch!

Girls who shave or remove all of the hair around their vaginal opening can also get skin infections, but more often, they develop skin irritation from vaginal discharge. See, when you have hair around the vaginal opening, it helps absorb and remove the discharge to keep it from sticking to your skin. Vaginal discharge has a pH (a chemistry thing) that can be irritating to the skin—more about that when we talk about the inside parts.

So the lesson here is that it's fine to trim any hair, anywhere. Trim means cut or shorten, *not* shave or remove completely.

Fuzzy?

What do you do with all that extra hair you get after puberty? The amount of hair you get will depend on your genetics. For instance, girls with Italian heritage will usually have more body hair, and girls from Asian descent may have very little body hair. Whatever your background, most girls have hair somewhere that they want to get rid of. What's safest? There are lots of hair removal products and procedures out there. Some are cheap, some are expensive, some work temporarily, some are permanent, some hurt and some don't. If you want to get rid of it, it's up to you to find the way that works best for you. Here is a table of the various ways to remove unwanted hair and some comments about each method. It may not include every method out there, but it will give you some information on the most common ones.

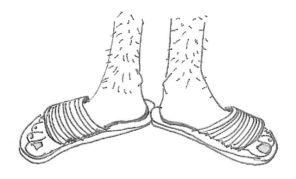

Method	How It Works	Things You Should Know
Tweezing or plucking	Use tweezers to pull individual hairs out by the root	Very inexpensive and easy Lasts longer than shaving Hurts a little depending on the area you are plucking
Shaving	Use a razor to remove hair	Inexpensive Easy and most common method of hair removal in the U.S. Works best if you shave skin that has been lubricated with soap or shaving cream/gel Temporary, sometimes requiring daily or twice daily use Hair that grows back is coarse Can cause skin irritation ("razor rash") or cuts; avoid this by using a clean, fresh razor and shaving hair in the same direction that it grows Can transmit diseases through sharing razor with someone else

Method	How It Works	Things You Should Know
Depilatories	Creams that are applied to the skin and unwanted hair; this dissolves the hair to the level of the skin	Easy and inexpensive May cause skin irritation Should not use around the vagina or on sensitive areas Some have an unpleasant odor Temporary
Waxing and other sticky gels or products that work by pulling hair out from the root	Warm or hot wax is applied over the unwanted hair and covered with a strip of cloth or paper; once the wax cools, the paper/cloth is quickly pulled off and pulls out all the hairs with it	Can do yourself (buy a "kit") or have it done at a spa or salon by a professional (more expensive) May cause minor skin burns, irritation or ingrown hairs Hurts as the hair is ripped off, but the pain is over with quickly Temporary, but lasts longer than shaving or depilatories

Method	How It Works	Things You Should Know
Prescription cream	Cream is applied to areas of unwanted hair twice a day every day	Requires a prescription from a medical professional and is only approved for use on the face Takes about 6 weeks to notice results Stops hair growth at the root as long as you use it every day; doesn't work unless you use it every day Expensive to use all the time
Electrolysis	A very small needle is inserted into each hair follicle, sending a mild electrical current that destroys the follicle; the hair is then pulled out with tweezers and hopefully won't grow back	Requires multiple treatments to remove all unwanted hair in an area Can be painful, but prescription numbing creams can help Expensive

Method	How It Works	Things You Should Know
Laser hair removal	A special type of laser or light is flashed from a device that is held over the area of unwanted hair, causing damage to the hair follicle so hair won't grow back out of it	Requires multiple treatments depending on the amount and location of hair Uncomfortable, but numbing creams can help Works best on darker hair Having a tan or sun exposure in the area will make it less effective and more difficult to get good results Can cause skin burns and scarring Safest and most effective when done by an experienced professional Can be very expensive
Bleaching	Bleaches dark hair blonde but doesn't remove hair	Works well for fine hair Is not a hair removal method, but just "camouflages" the hair that is bothersome Inexpensive and easy

The **Inside** Parts

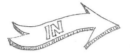

Your inside parts are obviously hard to see. Kind of like seeing your heart or lungs. We know they are in there, but don't expect to see them except in books or pictures. You'll just have to trust us on this one. Let's start on the outside and work our way to the innermost parts.

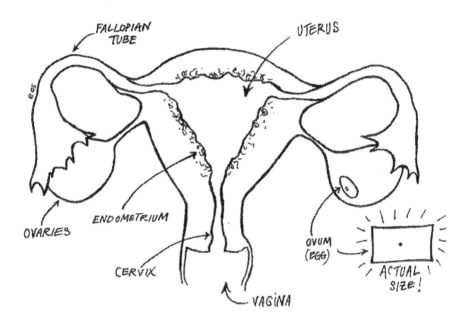

Vagina—the connection between your outside and inside parts. It is the passageway for menstrual blood, for sperm and for a baby at birth. It is a really cool body part for a couple of reasons (you think we're weird, don't you?). One, the vagina is very stretchy. If you put your finger in your vagina, you will notice that it is moist and wrinkly. It obviously needs to be stretchy for a baby to pass through it. The wrinkles or folds allow it to stretch more.

It's also really cool because it cleans itself (don't you wish your room could do that?). Clean may not be the first word that comes to mind about your vagina, but this is no joke. The vagina is cleansed constantly, and **vaginal discharge** is created as it cleans. This discharge will start to leak from the vagina around puberty. It is usually a white to yellowish liquid that will feel moist, sometimes wet. When it dries in your underwear, it will look more yellow and may feel kind of stiff or sticky. Don't panic—it's normal. As long as it doesn't stink, itch or change colors, it is normal.

Sometimes even normal discharge will make you feel itchy, especially if you don't have much **pubic hair** (whether it hasn't grown in yet or you've shaved it off). The pubic hair helps pull the discharge away from the skin, but if the discharge can't be pulled away from the skin, the moisture and pH (that chemistry thing) will cause the vulvar skin to get irritated and itchy. You can prevent this by using panty liners to help absorb the discharge or by using an ointment that contains zinc oxide (like a diaper rash cream—good for girls out of diapers, too!) around the vaginal opening. Okay. Enough vagina chat.

Cervix—at the inner end of the vagina is the cervix. It's like a very narrow two-way street, meaning it allows stuff to go in (sperm and some bacteria) or out (menstrual blood or baby). The opening is usually so small it can be considered "closed." That's why a tampon can't get lost in your body—the cervix acts as a dead end for the vagina. The cervix is also an amazing part of your body because it keeps a baby inside but then opens wide enough to let the baby pass through during birth. Wow.

Uterus—the womb or where a baby grows. It's a strong hollow muscle with a thick and lush lining that will allow a baby to grow! It is usually about the size of your fist, but can stretch and grow to hold a baby . . . some babies weigh up to 10 pounds or more (talk about Girl Power!). The uterus has three openings: the cervix that heads into the vagina (you already know about that one) and the other two, the right and left fallopian tubes that connect the uterus to the ovaries. These serve as the passageway for the egg (coming toward the uterus) and sperm (going into the fallopian tube to find the egg!). The fallopian tube openings are about the diameter of a hair, very tiny.

Endometrium—the lining of the uterus that is shed each month—as a period—if pregnancy does not occur. If pregnancy occurs, it's where the embryo (a fertilized egg) implants and starts to grow into a baby. It is a thick, lush lining that has a lot of nutrients, fluids and blood that are necessary to grow a baby.

Fallopian tubes—the tubes from the ovaries to the uterus that carry the egg once it is released (that's called *ovulation*). They are about three to four inches long on each side, and they are soft like a ribbon, not like a pipe. This is the place where the sperm and egg come together if fertilization occurs. Remember, the fallopian tubes are only as wide as a hair, so you can imagine how tiny the egg and sperm actually are! At the end of each fallopian tube is a fluffy opening called the *fimbria,* which are constantly but gently swishing over the ovaries to sweep the eggs into the tube. Visualize the gentle movement of a sea anemone. Can you feel your fimbriae swishing now? They are. Anyway, the inside of the tubes are made of special cells that continue the swishing to keep that egg moving in the right direction.

Ovaries—two oval things in the pelvis that are small, about the size of a medium strawberry. Each one is next to the fimbria of the fallopian tube. Girls are born with all the eggs they will ever have, which is way more than you could ever need! Can you believe we start off with millions? We save them up until puberty, then we only use one, maybe two, per month. Each egg is held in a small, fluid-filled sac called a *follicle*.

The Journey of the **Egg**

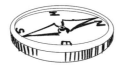

Now we've just listed everything in order from outside to inside, but if you think about how a pregnancy or periods happen, you have to think from inside to out.

Okay, shift to reverse gear. The pathway that an egg follows to find its way out begins at the ovaries; then once ovulation occurs (when the egg is released), it cruises and shimmies down a fallopian tube and lands nice and easy (plunk!) in the endometrium of the uterus. If it is not fertilized by a sperm, it will come out as a period (don't look for the actual egg, you'll never see it). If it is fertilized, a baby develops and is born about nine months later. Can you trace the path and name the parts as you go?

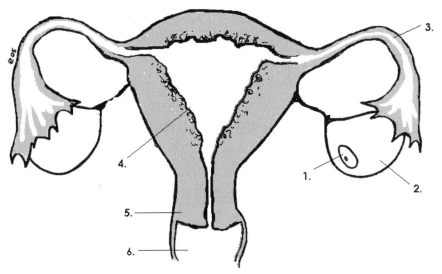

Answers:
1. follicle (or egg) 2. ovary 3. fallopian tube 4. endometrium 5. cervix 6. vagina

What about **Breasts**?!

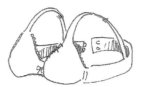

We can't forget our breasts! They deserve at least a little attention here. (Boys and the media certainly give them attention, so we will, too!)

You should know by now that they come in all shapes and sizes, and **no two are exactly alike,** including your two. Lopsided? Join the club. Most girls and women are, but it's not really that noticeable unless you are looking closely. If yours are more lopsided than you think they should be, check with your doctor.

Breasts have parts, too. The breast mound is the main part of your breast and is full of fatty tissue and glands that will produce milk. The nipple is the little bump in the center that can be indented, flat or poking out. Around the nipple is a circle of darker skin called the **areola** (uh REE oh luh). The areola or skin around it can be hairy, and the areola itself may have small white or light-colored bumps on it that are smaller than your nipple. Those extra bumps are gland openings—normal and nothing to worry about.

Nipples can have a mind of their own and suddenly become hard and even more obvious when you are cold, excited or anxious. It can be kind of embarrassing to some girls, but try not to worry too much about it. Just like everyone gets goose bumps when they are cold or nervous, your nipples can act like those goose bumps, too. Have you ever heard them called headlights? Party hats? It happens to all girls! Some girls like to wear bras to help with this occasional pop-up. Other reasons to wear a bra include comfort and general breast health. Bras may decrease the color and size of stretch marks and may help prevent back pains.

When should you start wearing a bra? Well, if you aren't already, it's up to you! Some women never wear a bra, and some don't go anywhere without one. Lots of girls start wearing a bra when their breasts show through their clothes or start to jiggle a little. When your breasts are growing, it's normal for them to be a little sore or sensitive. Sometimes wearing a bra can be more comfortable.

Your breasts will grow quickly before you start your period and then a little more after you start. During this growth phase, they may take on a shape that you don't like. Be patient, your breasts may continue to change shape and size up to about age 18. Because of this rapid growth, you may need to buy bras more often, because a properly fitted bra is important, especially when your breasts are growing. Bras can help prevent some stretch marks, but sometimes, no matter how much support you have for your breasts, those stretch marks happen anyway. It's genetic. **You can thank your ancestors!** Don't forget to buy a special sports bra for more physical activity. Finally, a bra will not prevent your breasts from becoming saggy later in life. That usually happens to some extent as we get older and is most noticeable after we have babies.

Breasts are another important part of your girlness for several reasons. They are sensitive when touched and can give us sexual pleasure (we'll talk about that more in chapter 8), but most importantly, breasts are for feeding babies. There is no food or formula that anyone can buy that is better for a baby than breast milk. And you know what? Your breast size has nothing to do with how much milk you can make. Even the smallest, pea-sized breasts can make enough milk to feed a big, hungry, chubby baby! Although most women can breast-feed, some decide not to for various personal or health reasons.

The **Rest** of Your Body

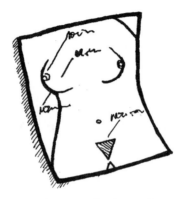

In case you haven't noticed, your body will grow a lot in middle school. It grows up some and out some, up some more, out some more. In the year before you start your period, you may grow three to four inches taller or more! After your period starts, you can still grow a little, but it is mostly in your trunk. Your legs, arms, feet, hands and head are all done by then!

Now what about that growing "out" part? Most girls complain about that part, but it is a part of getting that womanlike body. *Your whole shape will change, and it's for a good reason.* Your waist will be more obvious; your hips and thighs will grow larger. Sometimes your butt and hips will get bigger—and your breasts? Well, we've talked about them already. You are starting to look more like a teen or young woman—but remember, you're still a girl.

Take care of this new body you are growing. It has to serve you for a long, long, long, long time. Some of these changes are hard to accept, but remember that being a girl is a gift, and this new body is part of it!!!!!

Since We're Talking about **Girls**, We Gotta Talk about **BRAINS**!!

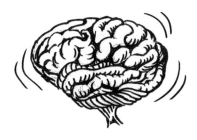

Finally, we can't leave out the most important part of your entire body . . . your brain! Your body's girl parts are not the only part of you getting a makeover once you start puberty. Inside that head of yours, there's a major construction zone! Your brain hasn't been this busy growing since you were a toddler! **Can you feel all the electricity, the power, the buzzing and whirling that's happening in there?** Thoughts, emotions, feelings, knowledge are all inside that head of yours. It is a busy place!

Believe it or not, your brain is largest around age eleven or twelve (and if you have a 12-year-old brother or sister, we're sure you'll have a hard time believing us!). But for brains, size doesn't matter much—it's the wiring that matters the most!

After age eleven or twelve, your brain starts to "delete" some of its unused parts and begin construction on some of the more grown-up parts. It takes a lot of time, and what you do, think and feel helps decide what parts to delete. It's kind of like deleting old files on your computer. Your brain is your computer, and if you leave some "files" unused for a long time, it starts to clean up and put away that old and outdated stuff.

At the same time it's cleaning out old files, your brain is also **figuring**

out how to do more complicated jobs. Scientists have given these jobs big words like "advanced reasoning," "abstract thinking" and "meta-cognition." (You can impress any adult with those words!) What that means is that your brain is becoming more and more able to think about things that you can't really see, like beliefs, trust and love. You become able to understand what it means to have choices and consequences. And your brain gets smarter every day!

You can also **think about "thinking."** That sounds weird, but when you were a little kid, you couldn't sit down and think about your own

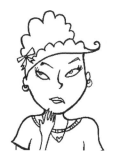

thoughts, analyze your feelings or think about how things affected you. Now you are beginning to do just that.

That's why friendships are meaning more to you—**you understand the feelings and emotional part of friends.** Friends are not just someone to "play" with anymore. They are people who *matter* to you because they make you feel good about who you are. Try explaining that to a seven-year-old, and you'll get a look or a grunt that says, "Huh?" instead of, "Oh yeah, I totally get it." But young teens do totally get it because their brains are growing just like they're supposed to. Get it?

These changes in your brain are also giving you some thoughts, ideas and emotions that are very common among teenagers. You may feel like you have people watching you sometimes, even though you know you really don't, like an imaginary audience. We don't mean you are crazy, hearing voices or feeling paranoid; you just feel like you are performing for others sometimes. It's okay. **That's helping you monitor your behaviors and think about how you act or want to act.** Sometimes it's good to "pretend" your parent or best friend is watching. It might keep you from doing something you really don't mean to do or shouldn't do.

You may also have **the [wrong] idea that bad things only happen to other people** and that you are invincible (that's a good vocabulary word—it means "it won't happen to me," "I can't be beat or hurt"). Think about, for example, getting seriously hurt on your bike. Most adolescents think, "I don't need to wear a goofy helmet because I'll never fall and hurt my head." But every year, hundreds of adolescents are killed or suffer permanent brain damage from falling off their bikes and hitting their heads. **And what about pregnancy?** Many teens have the idea that "it won't happen to me," so having sex without birth control is no big deal. That kind of thinking is why almost a MILLION teenage girls get pregnant *every year* in the United States, and one in four teen girls who has sex will get a sexually transmitted infection. That's right, one out of every four every year. Even though you may have feelings of being invincible—remember that bad things *can* happen, especially if you aren't being safe!

On a happier note, you also start **understanding justice and fairness better.** You start to understand why rules you may not like can still be important. You also begin to realize that the world is a big place, and you are a small part of it, but an important part that can help make it a *better* place.

Another area of your brain that is growing the fastest in adolescence has to do with emotions. That part also reacts to most of the hormones that are surging through your body. It's what makes you have lightning-fast emotions like we talked about in chapter 2, but it also makes **you look for activities and experiences that give you an emotional "high."**

What do we mean by "high"? Most people are talking about drugs when they use that word, but here it means when you get an amazingly awesome feeling from something.

Emotional highs come from all kinds of things, like singing, playing or listening to your favorite music, riding a dirt bike over a big ramp and catching a ton of air, rock climbing to a major height, galloping on a horse, Rollerblading as fast as you can go, riding a roller coaster, drawing a picture you love, laughing as loud as you can with friends who "get it" or writing a poem that other people appreciate.

Having an experience that gives you that awesome feeling doesn't have to be dangerous, but it usually does involve some risk . . . taking a chance either emotionally or physically. When you do that and succeed, you feel great. When you do that and don't succeed, it can hurt—either physically or emotionally.

Once you find something that gives you that great, awesome feeling, **practicing or spending time with that activity becomes important, especially in adolescence.** You become more skilled and familiar with the things that give you those awesome feelings. It's an important thing to experience in adolescence, and it's good for your brain development. Find something that makes you feel that way—a passion, a hobby, a challenge—and have fun!

Think of the things that give you that "emotional high" or make you feel good about yourself. Answer the questions below to help you figure out what these things are.

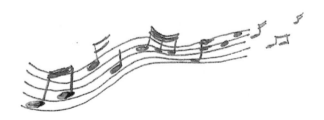

Things I love to do:

Things I do well:

Things I want to try or do more often:

Challenges I enjoy:

That's a **Wrap**

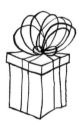

So can we quit with all this body talk? It's a ton of information. Promise—no quiz, but do you get it? This is a tough chapter, full of facts and new words. Feel free to move on. Come back to this chapter when and if you need to or if you ever just want to. It's here to help remind you about all the amazing stuff that is changing in you right now. It's also here to **reassure you that a lot of the "weird" stuff going on with your body is common to all preteen and teen girls.**

Just remember, all these changes in your body and brain take years to unfold and take hold. It's normal to feel totally freaked out, amazed, grossed out or excited by your body changes. **Some changes you will like; some you won't.** Over the years, your body will become comfortable again for you—like a pair of comfy, worn-in jeans. **Appreciate it for what it can do and what it will be able to do in the future.** It's an amazing, miraculous, awesome thing—you are wonderfully made, whether *you* think so right now or not!

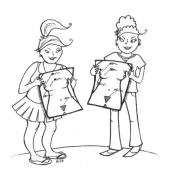

6

Periods, Period

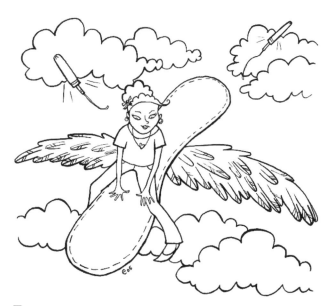

It's no secret that the whole reason we have periods is so that one day we can have babies. And having babies happens because of sex. So if we are going to talk about sex (which we are a lot), we have to talk about periods, first.

Having periods doesn't have much to do with sex, but if you decide to have sex, and most people do eventually, you better understand your periods very well! Even if you are not having sex for a long, long time, it's still important to understand the amazing events going on in your body that give you your little monthly "friend."

Blame It on Your **Hormones**

We bet you've heard women or girls complain about being "hormonal" or turning "emo" (emotional), or maybe you've heard your mom blame your moods on "raging hormones." Guess what? **Hormones are good things, not bad things.** They are chemicals made in our bodies that send messages or signals from one part to another. There are many, many different hormones circulating in each person's body. Two in particular are very involved in your menstrual cycle: estrogen and progesterone. Heard of them?

Like to **Cycle**?

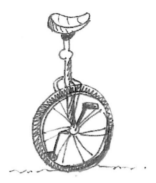

Your monthly cycle begins on the day you start your period. Hormones from the brain tell the ovary to start getting an egg ready. In the ovary, the egg grows in a little sac of fluid called a follicle. The follicle makes estrogen that causes the endometrium to grow a thick and lush lining. When the egg *ovulates* (which means it pops out of the ovary), the follicle then makes progesterone that prepares the endometrium for a pregnancy. If the egg is not fertilized by a sperm from a male, a pregnancy does not occur. With no pregnancy, the ovary stops making the progesterone, and that signals the endometrium to shed the lining (and that's a period). As the period begins, the brain signals the ovary to start over with a new follicle and a new lining in the endometrium. This amazing cycle then starts all over again!

Want the short report? Egg matures > egg ovulates > egg travels down fallopian tube and into the uterus. No pregnancy? Then the uterus recognizes that and sheds the old lining, which starts a period. Now that's an easier story to follow!

Another way to say it: It's kind of like a bed is made in the uterus for a baby to grow in. If there's no baby there, the uterus decides it's time to change the "bed," sort of like changing the sheets. How often do you change your sheets? In your uterus, it's once a month!

And even if you don't want it, here's the long report.

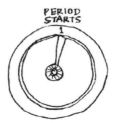

Cycle day 1. The first day you have menstrual bleeding is always considered day 1. It's usually anywhere from 25 to 35 days after your last period. Everyone always seems to think that period cycles are always 28 days or one month . . . but everyone is a little different, and cycles can be longer or shorter (anywhere from 21 to 45 days) and still be normal.

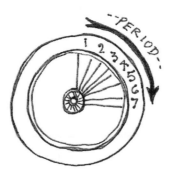

Cycle days 1–7. Periods usually last anywhere from three to seven days, but you only lose about two tablespoons of actual blood in all that time. It seems like more doesn't it? That's because of the other fluids and tissue that are released (think of them as the pillow cases and bedspread that need to be cleaned, too). Your bleeding is happening because there is no pregnancy, and the uterus has decided to release the old lining and begin a new lining (change the sheets!). Your uterus pushes out the period (old sheets) by contracting its muscular walls. Some girls will feel these contractions as cramps.

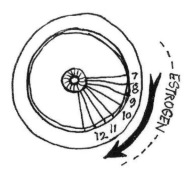

Cycle days 7–12. At the same time that you are having your period, your brain and ovaries are already talking. Your brain is recruiting another egg for the next cycle, and your uterus is getting orders to prepare a fresh lining. Your hormones are helping with all this communication. The follicle (which holds the recruited egg) in your ovary is making that hormone called estrogen that helps thicken the lining of the uterus. So as soon as your bleeding is done, your uterus is already "fluffing up the sheets," or getting a new lining ready for the next cycle in case an embryo is on the way.

Now for this whole thing about babies. Your body needs a lot of practice with its cycles before it's really ready for a baby. That's why you start your periods way before you are ready to actually have sex and get pregnant.

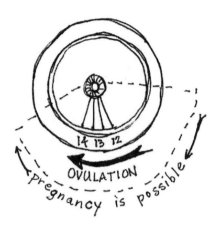

Cycle days 12–14. Ovulation time. Now that the next egg has been recruited, it is ready for take off. The follicle that it has been growing in will open up and let it go! This is called *ovulation.* Some girls actually feel a slight twinge or cramp when this happens. If there is discomfort, it's called *mittelschmerz* (dare you to use that in your next English paper!!). That's a German word that means "middle pain." Most girls are clueless that such an amazing thing is happening in there.

This is the time when you may also notice that your vaginal discharge seems a little more watery or slimey. This happens because your hormones tell your cervix to change the discharge to make it easier for sperm to pass through. The cervix says okay, and makes the discharge extra slippery. Pregnancy can happen during about eight days every cycle. The six or seven days before and two or three days after ovulation are the days that pregnancy is most likely to happen if you are having sex. **Because ovulation is unpredictable and young girls' cycles are not always the same every month, it is really hard to figure out exactly when pregnancy can or can't happen.**

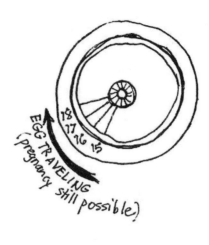

Cycle days 15–18. Ovulation has usually happened by now, and the egg is still traveling down the tube. If it has already hooked up with a sperm, an embryo is forming (we'll talk about that more in chapters 6 and 7). Most likely, it's alone and enjoying the massage as it is swished down the fallopian tube into the uterus. Once the egg arrives in the uterus, it hangs out for a couple days before it's time to go.

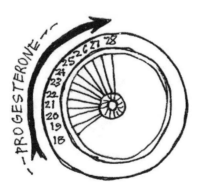

Cycle days 18–28 or so. This is a time for rest in the endometrium. The follicle that had released the egg is now making a new hormone called progesterone. Progesterone will make the fluid in the cervix thicken and will get the lining in tip-top shape in case an embryo arrives. If there is no pregnancy in the uterus, the amount of progesterone falls and the endometrium can't live without it, so it leaves the uterus as a period, which brings you back to day 1.

As the progesterone levels are changing, some girls get moody or might feel more hungry than usual. Acne can worsen during this time. Some girls even feel a little puffy or bloated. That's why you might hear girls complaining when they're about to get their periods. All these symptoms are common and go away as soon as a period starts. Rarely, these symptoms are so bad that they affect your friendships and relationships at home. If that happens with you, please talk with your doctor because there are things that can help.

What if My Periods Are Not Regular?

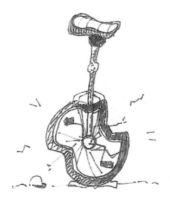

Let's back up a little. After your very first period (it's called *menarche,* which sounds like anarchy and is pronounced MEN ar kee), you might have another period a month later, or it might not come again for several months.

After your first few periods, you should expect your periods to occur anywhere from 21 to 45 days apart. It might be 28 days one month, 40 days the next, 32 days the next. That's all normal at first. A period doesn't always come at the same exact time every month (remember months aren't all the same length, either), but **it should start to show a predictable pattern within a few years after you start.**

If fact, the age you are at menarche can predict how soon your periods will start happening in a regular pattern.

Age at Menarche	Years until Very Predictable Periods
Under 11	1 to 2 years
11 to 12	Up to 2 or 3 years
Over 12	Up to 4 or 5 years

Periods will become "very" predictable once you start ovulating regularly. It's not as reliable as the TV schedule or even as the trash pickup days, but it's as reliable as they can get—that means within two to three days of the predicted time. Remember, *to ovulate* means to release an egg from your ovary. Once you start to ovulate with every cycle, then your periods become predictable. Your period will always start about 14 to 16 days *after* you ovulate. Problem is, you don't always know when to expect ovulation. Like we said before, most girls have no clue when they ovulate because they usually don't feel it. But if your periods are happening *about* the same number of days apart every time, you can know that you are probably ovulating. **Miraculous!**

So far we've been talking about regular ovulation, which means you are ovulating pretty much every month. But did you know **you can**

ovulate before you even get your first period? After that, some of your cycles will include ovulation and some won't. That means pregnancy can happen before a girl even has her first period if she is having sex.

Menstrual Calendar

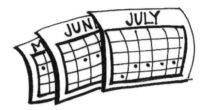

Keep up with your periods by using the boxes below whenever you have bleeding. Copy it or make a chart like it to keep track of your bleeding—the heavier your bleeding is, the darker you fill in the box. Very light days (some people call this "spotting") can be shown with just a dot in the box for that date. If you develop any irregular bleeding, this chart or one like it will be very helpful to your doctor. Besides, it will also help you recognize the pattern of your periods and help you predict when you will have your next one.

Predicting Your Periods

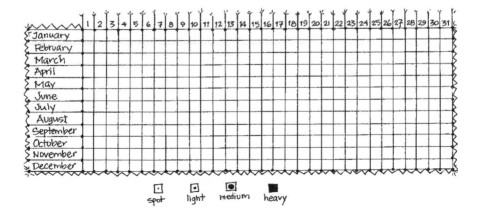

By keeping track of your periods on a calendar, you can usually tell when you should expect your next period. To calculate your *cycle length,* look at the past few periods on your calendar. Starting with the *first day* of a period, count the number of days until the *first day* of the next period. Do this for two or three cycles.

Most cycles will be between 21 and 45 days long. If your cycle length is about the same (within three to five days of each other) for several cycles, you can then start predicting your next periods pretty accurately.

If your periods are completely irregular, check the table on page 117 to see if it is time for you to be ovulating regularly yet. If it is, and you are still having unpredictable periods, talk with your doctor. Also, if your periods are skipping more than two months at a time, you should talk with your doctor. Some girls and women never ovulate regularly and may need medication to make their periods predictable.

How Much Bleeding Is Normal?

Most periods have only a couple tablespoons to about one-half cup of blood and fluid . . . and it's mostly fluid and tissue, not blood. That's why it doesn't always look like real blood, but instead looks kind of brown or dark maroon, even blackish. Our bodies can make up for that amount of blood loss in no time, so we do not become **anemic** (have a low blood count).

As we've mentioned, most periods last anywhere from three to seven days. It is normal to have heavier blood flow in the first one or two days, then it gets lighter toward the end. The number of pads or tampons that are normal to use will depend on how soaked you let them become and what types you are using.

Clots are dark clumps of blood that are the consistency of liver or old Jello-O. Clots happen when blood stays in one place for a while, like in your vagina. You are most likely to see clots in the morning from the menstrual blood that has been in your vagina while you were lying down. When you get up, you might pass small clots. If you use a tampon, you might also see clots hanging on to the end of it when you take it out. These are normal, but if you have a lot of larger clots, that could signal heavier-than-normal bleeding.

Cramps!

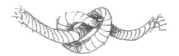

Some girls will have cramping in their lower abdomen or pelvis before or during their periods. Sometimes the pain is even in the vulva, upper thighs or lower back. Most older teens and women will have at least some mild discomfort with their periods. About 10 percent (one in ten, right?) will have severe cramps that make them stop doing activities they would normally do.

Menstrual cramping happens because the uterus (made of muscle tissue) squeezes to release the tissue and blood that make up your period. The squeezing is caused by that hormone (progesterone) and some other chemicals (called *prostaglandins*) that are released after ovulation.

If you feel bloated (full or puffy in your lower belly) or crampy with your periods, there are some things you can do to feel better:

- **Exercise**, such as walking, jogging, swimming, bicycling, stretching or yoga. These things really do help cramps . . . we're not kidding!
- **Take essential fatty acids** (especially omega-3) supplements like flaxseed oil, evening primrose oil or fish oil tablets.
- **Avoid red meat** and fried, fatty or greasy food (they have saturated fats, which can actually increase cramping).
- **Try medications**, such as ibuprofen 400 to 600 milligrams every six to eight hours or naproxen 440 milligrams every twelve hours. These may sound like big names you've never heard, but there are brand names that you are probably more familiar with. You'll have to look at medication labels to see what is really in them. These doses are a little higher than the instructions on the bottle advise, but they are closer to prescription doses often used for menstrual cramps. It's safe to use these doses for a couple of days. These medications block the prostaglandins that cause cramps and usually work better than some products that say they are for menstrual cramps, including aspirin or acetominophen. Aspirin products usually do little for cramps and may make bleeding heavier. Some medicines for cramps even contain caffeine. Caffeine does nothing for menstrual cramps and might make breast tenderness worse. Read the labels on medications you can buy without a prescription to find out exactly what is in them! Check with a parent before you take any type of medication.
- **A heating pad or a warm bath** always feels nice.

If you have tried the things above and still have cramps that stop you from doing things or make you miss school, you should **talk with your doctor.** There are prescription medications and hormones that can treat even the most severe cramps. There are also some medical conditions that can cause bad cramps. Your doctor can discuss these with you and make sure you are okay.

Period Supplies

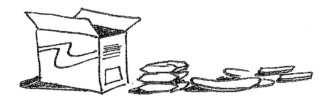

When you have your period, you obviously need to use pads or tampons (affectionately known, in totally unhip terms, as **feminine hygiene products**) to keep the blood off your clothes. There are *tons* of different brands in *tons* of different shapes and sizes. After a few periods, you'll know what works best for you.

Whether you use pads or tampons, you should change them at *least* every four to six hours and may need to change them more frequently if your menstrual flow is heavy. If you aren't familiar with them, here are some of the products out there. If you know all this . . . feel free to skip it and move on!

Pads

Pads are made with an adhesive that attaches to the crotch of your underwear. Just unwrap the pad, pull off the strip that covers the adhesive and put the pad in your underwear (sticky side against your underwear, not YOU! Ouch!). Adjust the pad into place as you pull your underwear up. There are different types of pads to choose from, including:

Pantyliner. This is a really thin pad that works for very light flow. Some girls like to use a pantyliner when they are also using a tampon, just in case they overflow the tampon. Some girls also like to use these for the vaginal discharge they have between periods.

Minipad. A little thicker than the pantyliner, this is for light to normal flow.

Maxipad. This one can feel pretty thick. Some girls say it feels like a diaper! It's good for heavy flow days or at night because it can absorb a lot.

"Wings." Pads with "wings" have flaps on the sides that you wrap around the crotch of your underwear. Sometimes a lot of running or activity will make your pad bunch up in the middle so that your menstrual flow goes over the edge and stains your underwear. The wings can help prevent that.

Sanitary napkins. Another term for menstrual pads, it usually refers to maxis.

Reusable pads. Some girls and women choose to use cotton pads that they can wash and reuse. They are probably better for the environment because you are not using disposable products. You can find them at health food stores.

Tampons

Tampons are little padlike things that actually go inside your vagina to absorb the menstrual flow as it comes out of the cervix. Sounds painful, but really, if you put it in right, you won't even feel it!

You put tampons in with an **applicator** that helps you insert the tampon into the vagina. There is also a brand that doesn't have an applicator, so you just put it in with your finger. The box they come in will have directions—look at the pictures they provide, and it will help. Just like pads, tampons come in a variety of sizes. For your first time, it definitely helps to use the slender or "light" size tampons. Sometimes it helps to put your finger in your vagina first to see what direction you need to "aim" the tampon. All tampons have a **string** on them so you can just pull the string to take the tampon out when it is time to change it. *Don't worry,* the strings don't break!!!! Even if they did, the vagina is a "dead end," so a tampon **cannot get lost inside you** and end up coming out of your nose! (Whew!)

Tampons are nice because you can swim and do other activities with them and not have to worry about having a bulky pad on. Can you imagine trying to wear a pad in a bathing suit and then getting it wet in the pool?

It is safe to use tampons even with your first period. Some girls, though, feel more comfortable trying their first tampon after they are a little more used to having periods. When you decide to use a tampon for the first time, make sure you are on your period with a pretty normal to heavy flow. This is because the tampon comes out a lot easier when it is soaked. If it is dry, it feels like you are tugging on the walls of the vagina . . . ouch! **There is no reason to "practice" using a tampon** before you are on your period. It will work, but it takes a little getting used to.

If your mom doesn't want you to use a tampon, you should ask why. Tampons have only been around for a couple of generations, so a lot of women your mom's age or grandmother's age were told they couldn't use tampons until they were married. This means they couldn't use tampons until after they had sex. **Tampons won't break your hymen, injure your vagina or tarnish your reputation as a nice girl.** Even the super-plus size tampons are a lot smaller than an erect penis! And since you put a tampon in yourself, you will know how much pressure you can apply to get it in without hurting yourself.

Another reason some people are scared of using tampons is a problem called **toxic shock syndrome (TSS).** TSS became well known when it started happening among women who used one particular brand of tampons that is no longer made. Toxic shock syndrome is a severe infection with a particular type of bacteria, and it is only rarely associated with tampon use. (It's actually more common with surgery or skin infections.) Recently, it has occurred a little more frequently because of super absorbent brands. If you use one of these make sure you remove it within four-six hours. So the bottom line is that tampons are safe to use if used properly.

How do you use them properly? Well, if you are using tampons, just as with pads, you'll need to change them regularly. If your flow is heavy, you'll know to change your tampon when you feel it starting to leak. If your flow is light, use a light or thin tampon, and don't wear it longer than six hours. If you forget to take one out and leave it in for several days, you'll remember when you start to notice a horrible odor or start having spotting that has a bad odor. An old, bloody tampon that sits in a vagina for several days will cause just that. Yuck! Hold your nose, take it out and wrap it up in something that will contain the smell! It happens. Just let it be a lesson: What goes in, must come out!

PMS?

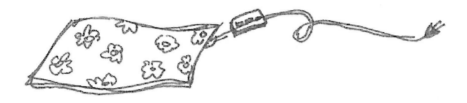

Some teens and women notice changes in the way they feel before their period. Symptoms can start anywhere in the one to two weeks before your period starts. They might include emotional things like crying easily, being moody or grumpy, or wanting to be alone. They can also be physical things like breast soreness, cramping, feeling puffy or craving certain foods.

When these types of feelings affect the things you do or your relationships with your friends or family, it's called PMS (it stands for **premenstrual syndrome**)—it's a real medical diagnosis, **not an excuse**. Sometimes people want to blame anger or emotions on PMS, but it may just be real anger or real emotions. There's a little good news since PMS *won't* happen at all unless you are ovulating regularly (remember that can take several years after you start!).

If you think you have PMS, you can do some things to make it better. First, you can predict when you will start your period and then also predict when your PMS will start. Use the menstrual calendar we provided. If you are prepared for it, it may not affect you so much.

PMS Busters

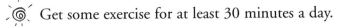 Get some exercise for at least 30 minutes a day.

Eat a dinner that is rich in complex carbohydrates, low in protein and fat—especially avoid animal protein and fat.

Avoid caffeine and salty foods.

Make sure you get some alone time to relax: Write in your journal, listen to some music or just do nothing!

Taking certain vitamins and minerals may help, including vitamin B_6 tablets, calcium, magnesium and vitamin E.

Taking omega-3 fatty acids, like evening primrose oil, fish oil or flaxseed oil, can help with mood problems, cramping and breast tenderness.

Wearing a supportive bra like a sports bra can help with breast tenderness.

Drinking herbal diuretic, caffeine-free tea can help with the bloating or puffiness. Remember to drink plenty of water!

Only about three or four in one hundred women will have PMS that's so bad they need medications to help it. That is rare. If you think you have PMS that is really bad, your doctor should be able to help you with medications or other suggestions.

Do Something **Special** for Yourself

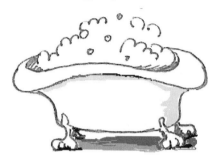

Lots of women think that periods are a real burden. Some even call their period "the curse"! But that's not necessarily how it has to be. In fact, most girls and women don't let periods get in their way at all.

Some people will also say, "Oh, you're a woman now." Guess what? Not! **There's a lot more to being a woman than just having a period.** You are still a girl, and you can still have all the fun that girls are supposed to have. Don't let your period get in your way!

If you find yourself feeling crabby or crampy around your period time, use it as a signal for you to do something nice for yourself, something you love . . . alone! Like to read? Play music? Watch the clouds? Curl up with your pet? Do it! Enjoy something special that gives you YOU TIME, and it will automatically make you feel a little better! You can use this time to focus on yourself. You may find that you actually enjoy and look forward to doing something special for yourself, even if it is period time. We hope that girls with Girl Power will celebrate their gift of girlhood, and having a period is just part of what makes all of us sisters special.

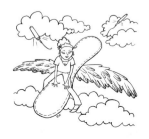

Boy, Oh Boy!

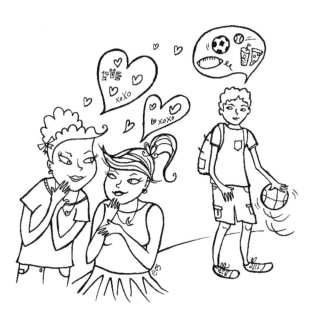

Enough about periods for a while, let's talk about boys!

Now, for this whole thing about having babies—it won't happen just because you have a period. It takes sperm from a man getting together with an egg from a woman to make a baby. Funny thing about guys is that they don't start making sperm until they go through puberty. (Remember, we are born with all of our eggs. Guys have to start from scratch.)

So have you noticed your guy friends going through puberty? Girls go through it several years earlier than guys. You are probably already in the midst of it, but your **guy friends are just noticing changes around ages eleven to fourteen.** That's partly why girls are sometimes "romantically interested" long before their guy friends are clued in to girls and crushes.

You'll know they are catching up in the puberty scene when you notice some thin, whispy hair on their upper lips (trying to become a mustache). You might notice more acne, voice changes and fast increases in their height. What you don't notice is one of their first signs of puberty. Their testicles enlarge and their penises grow (getting more information than you want?). It seems unfair that one of the first signs of puberty for a girl is obvious to everyone (we start growing breasts, and it's hard to hide that!). For guys this early sign is not so obvious (well, that's probably a good thing!).

Boy Parts

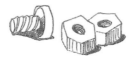

Well, we have to talk about it a little, so in case you didn't know yet, a boy's "private body parts," or external genitalia, are different from yours, especially in one area (no kidding!). Here are the words:

Penis (also known as a dick, a pecker, a unit, a johnson, a tally wacker, a weenie, a prick, a one-eyed monster . . . why so many names?!)— the tubelike thing that boys pee out of. It's also where sperm comes out. It's made of soft spongy tissue and is usually soft and floppy. When a guy gets sexually excited, the spongy tissue becomes full of blood (engorged). This makes the whole penis hard, and it "stands up" instead of flopping down—that's called an **erection** (or a hard-on, a woody, a boner). The penis needs to be erect to allow it to go into the vagina during sex. An erection is an interesting thing . . . really! So interesting, in fact, that we have more about it in the erection section later in this chapter . . . keep reading!

Urethra—connects the bladder (which is where urine is stored) to the penis and outside, so it's **where the urine (pee) comes out.** It is also connected with the parts **involved in sperm travel.** That means it's how the sperm gets out, too. It contains a valve that is like a door that lets only one of these things happen at a time. So when a guy is peeing, sperm can't come out, and likewise, when sperm is coming out, he can't pee. When we get more into the sex stuff later, this will seem more important!

Testes (also called testicles)—where guys make sperm and where the male hormone (called *testosterone*) comes from. Testosterone is the hormone that causes boys to grow facial hair, pubic hair, larger muscles and thickened vocal cords that give them their deeper voice (after it goes through the squeaky phase while the voicebox is growing). Guys have two testes, and they often call them their "balls" or their "nuts." They can be really tender and painful if hit or bumped hard. That's why guys in sports have to wear a plastic guard called an athletic cup over their penis and testicles to protect those sensitive parts. Some guys in other sports may wear a **jock strap,** which holds the penis and testicles close to the body and keeps them from flopping and swinging too much. A jock strap keeps a guy's privates comfortable and secure, like a jogging bra keeps our breasts snug and comfy during vigorous activity.

Scrotum—the sac of skin that hold the testicles. It's located behind the penis and between the legs. Did you know that sperm can only be made properly at a temperature that is slightly lower than our usual body temperature (in fact, they grow best at precisely 96.6 degrees Fahrenheit)? That's why the scrotum hangs away from the body and keeps the testicles cooler, so they can do their thing. In really cold weather, the scrotum will pull closer into the body to keep the testicles at the right temperature. So guys kind of have this built-in incubator with its own thermometer . . . wow! But don't believe for a minute that hanging out in a hot tub will kill a guy's sperm and make it impossible to get pregnant!

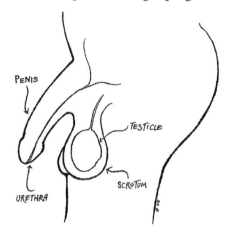

Sperm—the little things that a male makes that fertilize a female's egg. Sperm are so tiny that millions of them would fit into a teaspoon. You can't see a sperm unless you look under a microscope. If you do that, they actually look like tiny tadpoles, and they swim!

It takes about 90 days for a sperm to grow and mature in the male. When they come out of the penis, it is called **ejaculation**. For girls, only one egg is released each cycle, but for a guy, each time he ejaculates, he lets go of **many millions of sperm**. Some sperm will make girl babies, and some will make boy babies, so it's up to the man's sperm, not the woman's egg, to determine whether a baby boy or baby girl will be made. (By the way, the plural form of sperm is sperm. So it's one sperm, two sperm, five million sperm.)

Epididymus—a *very* long, coiled-up tube on the outside surface of each testicle. It's where the baby sperm spend a few weeks while they are growing into mature sperm . . . **kind of like the incubator.** When a male ejaculates, the sperm come from the epididymus, travel through some tubes and go out the opening at the end of the penis.

Prostate and seminal vesicles—two glands that are inside a male that add **fluid** to the sperm so they have something to swim in and **nutrition** for the trip (have snacks, will travel!). Once the fluid is added to the sperm, the mixture is called semen.

Semen—we just told you what this is, but we want to make sure you realize that semen is what comes out of the penis during sex or sexual excitement (the act is called ejaculation or "coming," and the fluid itself is called **semen, ejaculate** or **cum**). When it comes out, it amounts to less than a tablespoon of liquid, but guess how many sperm are in it? MILLIONS!!! And it only takes ONE to fertilize an egg! When ejaculation happens, all those little sperm race to see which one can get to the egg first and make a baby. Talk about competitive!

Erection Section

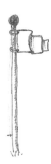

If you are like most girls, erections seem like a really unusual phenomenon to you. For a girl, the closest thing that happens like that and can be noticeable to others is when you are wearing a thin shirt and your nipples get hard and poke out like headlights coming on! Sometimes embarrassing, sometimes not even noticeable. For guys, erections can be even worse.

Can you imagine something between your legs suddenly becoming hard, about twice its usual size and sticking up? That's the embarrassing thing that happens to boys when they are in puberty and beyond. Boys can get erections even as babies. It happens sometimes if they have to pee or if they rub or play with their penises. In puberty, boys get "boners" a lot more frequently because of their hormones. Erections can be **unpredictable and can happen at the worst times** . . . like when a guy is asked to get up in front of the class to read a report. Yikes.

Erections usually happen if a guy is thinking about something sexy or having a fantasy. It will also happen if he is "playing with himself" or masturbating. The embarrassing part for guys, though, is that **sometimes they have no control** over a sudden erection. It's certainly *not* something you want to point out to them like, "Um, excuse me, is that a banana in your pocket or are you having an erection?"

Most of the time, guys find a way to hide it. They either won't stand up, or they might put their hands in their pockets to hold themselves down. ("Down boy, down!") Sometimes they will think about something *un*exciting (like kissing their grandmothers) to make erections go away. These erections usually last only a minute or so when they happen like that.

A teen guy will almost definitely get an erection if he is dancing closely, body to body, with his "sweetie" or if his crush sits on his lap. If you are the subject of one of these erections, don't worry, ***it's not your responsibility to help him make it go away.*** Some guys might expect you to "do something" sexual to help them "finish" their sexual excitement with an orgasm (read more about that in the next section). The great news here is that ALL guys know how to take care of that all by themselves. You should feel NO obligation, and don't let any guy tell you differently!

The other thing you might hear about is a nocturnal emission—fondly known as a *wet dream*. A wet dream is when a guy ejaculates in his sleep. It might happen because of a sexy dream, or it might just happen for no reason. No need to ask your guy friends about it. They won't want to talk about it, and some guys never have one.

The **Journey** of a Sperm

If you've been paying attention, we are sure you know that sex is how a baby is made, and we will definitely talk a lot more about sex stuff in this book. For now, let's concentrate on getting this anatomy straight. It seems like a lot to learn, but it makes more sense when you understand how it all connects and works together. Let us take you on an **amazing, swirly, twisty-turny journey** that will start with a sperm and end with a pregnancy happening in a female. Ready? Here we go.

- Sperm are made in the **testes.** (You know that by now, right?)
- They travel into the **epididymus** (incubator), where they hang out for a few weeks until they grow and mature.
- With sexual excitement (we'll get to that later), they are pushed through another tube called the **vas deferens.** In the vas deferens, they pass the *seminal vesicles* and *prostate gland* where they pick up their nutrients and fluids (snacks) and officially become semen.
- As the journey out continues, the sperm travel into the penis ,and with **ejaculation,** the semen squirts out of the penis through the **urethra.**
- If they come out during **sexual intercourse,** they find themselves in a woman's vagina (hey, where are we? how'd we get here?). And they're off, up the vagina, through the **cervix,** into the **uterus,** then into one of the fallopian tubes. Little do they know, there is usually only one egg. So that means about HALF of them will make a wrong turn down the empty **fallopian tube** (you know how men don't like to ask for directions. . . .).

- Anyway . . . ahoy! After a long upstream swim, some (actually many many thousands) of the sperm finally reach the egg that has been floating peacefully down the fallopian tube since it ovulated. Eggs only live about 24 to 48 hours after ovulation, but sperm can live up to a week, so timing is important.

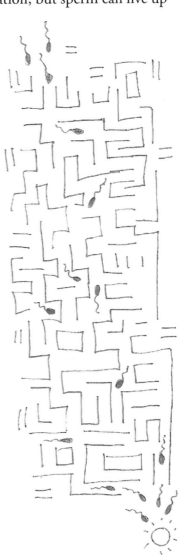

- They all surround the egg and start wiggling their way into it. Once one sperm gets through the egg's wall, a special chemical is released that prevents any others from getting in. It's like a lock down (or getting grounded!).

- The egg and sperm, now together, will share their genes (DNA or biological information that determines how a person looks, grows, etc.), and they begin to grow into a ball of cells that can eventually become a baby. The ball of cells (called an *embryo*) will then travel back into the uterus. It settles into the thick, lush, nutrient-rich endometrium (remember the "bed"?).

- Blood vessels from the mother begin to feed the pregnancy, and it continues to grow for the next nine months into a real, live baby! The birth of that baby is another story we don't have space for in this book, but it is incredible!

It's an amazing miracle!

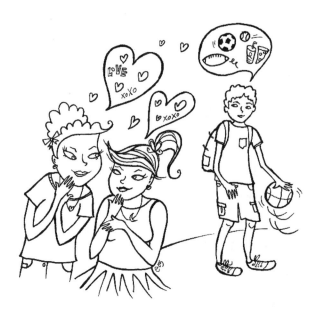

S-E-X

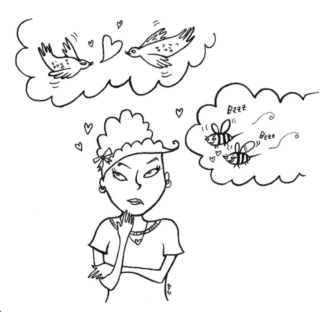

When you hear the word *sex*, what do you think of? Your parents or grandparents may refer to sex as "the birds and the bees." Whatever. Most people think of that penis-in-vagina thing, but there's really **a lot more to it.** What about feeling attracted to someone? Holding hands? Kissing? Touching? Intercourse?

Oral sex? All of these are part of sex. And the penis-in-vagina thing is usually near the end, not the beginning, of sex. See? There's a lot to talk about when we say that very big little three-lettered word, S-E-X.

Sex: The Basics

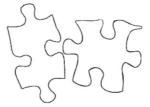

Let's start with the basics. From a scientific viewpoint, pregnancy is just a sperm and an egg coming together at just the right time to make a new living creature. For many animals, that's about all there is to it. You might see frogs mating in your backyard (maybe you just thought they were playing piggyback). You probably have seen a dog trying to mate with another dog (or sometimes someone's leg). **But for humans, who have the unique ability to feel love, to communicate, to bond with other humans and to express feelings, sex is a *much* bigger deal!** It should involve a lot of emotional closeness and intimacy, a lot of trust and comfort. It should be something that *both* people are ready for and agree to do.

Puberty is when your body becomes sexually mature. But to be mature enough for responsible sexual activity is another whole long and involved process that includes your emotions, your sense of self and your ability to be in a healthy relationship. **Just because you have the parts and the plumbing doesn't mean you're ready to use them** (more about this later).

There are a lot of ways to safely explore your body's feelings and pleasures besides having sex. There's other stuff, like "petting" or making out, before "going all the way." Girls with Girl Power need to know about the basics of sex, but they also know that Empowered Girls wait until they are mature enough to deal with all the responsibilities and consequences that come with sex. They don't have sex before they KNOW they are ready.

The actual "activity" of sexual intercourse can sound sort of icky and awkward, but in the right relationship, when there is love and trust and comfort, it is not icky at all. Bear with us while we explain a few details. (Here comes the birds and the bees part you've been waiting for!)

Birds and the Bees?

What do they have to do with sex? Great question. It all goes back to Victorian times when sex was never mentioned, and people were so uptight about sex that they made up an explanation for reproduction based on plants in nature. The birds were part of plant reproduction because they spread seeds. They would eat berries and seeds, then spread them as they left their droppings throughout nature. That's the birds' part. The bees then were responsible for helping things in nature to grow by pollinating them. So the Victorian families gave that explanation about seeds and pollination to help explain sex to their "children." That explanation usually occurred on the eve of their weddings. Talk about some confusion!! Aren't you glad we're just getting this sex stuff all out in the open?

Foreplay

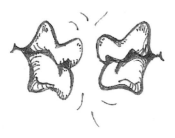

When a couple is sexually excited, they may kiss and touch each other. **It feels good physically and emotionally.** Usually, their hearts beat fast, they start breathing more heavily and they may also get sweaty. As a man gets sexually excited, he will get an erection. As the woman gets sexually excited, her vagina will make extra liquid (it's called lubrication) that makes the vagina more slippery. The vagina will also start to expand some and become more elastic or stretchy. Her nipples and clitoris may also get hard or erect. All this excitement and touching or caressing is called foreplay. It prepares the man's body and the woman's body for sexual intercourse, but sexual intercourse doesn't HAVE to happen just because there is sexual excitement.

Now to That Penis-in-Vagina Thing

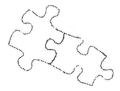

Sex can happen in lots of different "positions," but usually the woman is on the bottom and the man is on the top and they are facing each other. The man's erect penis is inserted into the woman's vagina. It seems like that might take some awkward positioning, but we fit together in this way like two puzzle pieces. Once the penis is inside her vagina, the couple will move their bodies to make the penis move in and out or back and forth because it feels good for both of them. The in-and-out movement feels good on the penis for the man and also feels good on the vagina and clitoris for the woman. The closeness also feels good emotionally if both are relaxed and wanting to do what they're doing.

As the sex continues, the excitement builds to the point where an **orgasm** may occur. For a man, an orgasm is when ejaculation occurs. Before ejaculation, there is a small amount of fluid (called pre-ejaculate or pre-cum) that leaks out of the penis and may contain sperm. So sperm can be present even if ejaculation has not occurred. And remember, it only takes ONE sperm to get pregnant. After the male ejaculates, the penis gets soft again, and he can't have another orgasm until he gets another erection.

For a woman, orgasm is less obvious on the outside (and it doesn't usually involve all the crazy screaming you see on TV or in the movies), but she feels a strong and pleasurable physical reaction through her whole body. Some women can have more than one orgasm during sex, but most don't.

We're making it sound pretty unexciting and scientific here, but **sex, in the right setting with the right person, is an amazing and wonderful connection.** Don't think from this simple description that it isn't really special.

Like a **Virgin**

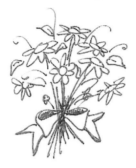

Lots of teens AND adults pay a lot of attention to the word *virgin*. In the truest sense of the word, a virgin is a person (male or female) who is sexually "pure." That means she or he has never had sex. But as you'll learn throughout this book, there's a lot more to sex than just a penis in a vagina. Is a girl still a virgin if she has oral sex? Some teens think they are still "technically" a virgin even if they are doing some pretty outrageous sexual things as long as a penis doesn't go in the vagina. How "pure" is oral or anal sex? Although it might prevent pregnancy, infections can still be a big risk. As far as we're concerned, the word *virgin* doesn't hold much significance medically because "technical virgins" are still at risk for infections and the emotional consequences of sex. The meaning of *virgin* is deeper than a "technical" definition; it involves purity of the mind as well as the body, and it's something that you have control over. Just don't try to fool yourself into thinking "technical virginity" is risk free. Face the truth and protect yourself from the consequences. We'll discuss what those risks are later in this chapter.

The **Big** O
(We don't mean Oprah, but we love her anyway.)

Orgasms feel great, no question. And lots of people make a huge deal out of them. It's important to understand that sometimes orgasm doesn't happen at all during the penis-in-vagina part of sex, particularly for women. Most women need to feel very relaxed, comfortable and safe to experience orgasm. **Sex isn't just about orgasm,** and it can still feel good even if an orgasm doesn't happen. Being sexual with someone you love is about expressing warmth, closeness and intimacy—an orgasm is an added bonus.

Sometimes for guys, orgasm (ejaculation) may happen very quickly and actually before they are ready for it to happen. Teenage boys in general are not always able to control how long they can keep an erection. That means a guy can get an erection and ejaculate **before a girl even starts to get sexually aroused** and enjoy the experience—that can lead to frustration. For a lot of women, sex is more about emotional attachment, comfort and security in a relationship. Guys sometimes get a reputation for being just into the act without the emotional attachment. There are definitely some great guys out there who are looking for emotional intimacy before sexual intimacy. There are also guys, especially teen guys, who can seem unemotional and pushy when it comes to sex. It's not always the guys, though. There are also girls who are pushy and unemotional when it comes to doing sexual things. For too many teens, it seems to be more about bragging rights and being able to say, "Hey, I got laid!" Just remember, sex isn't supposed to be like a Nike ad. It's about a lot more than "just doing it."

Solo Sex

Orgasm can happen without sexual intercouse. It can happen for males and females just from sexual touching or even in sexual dreams. A lot of males and females will touch themselves sexually. This can just feel good, or it can be intense enough to create an orgasm. Touching yourself sexually is called **masturbation**. When guys masturbate, they will hold and rub their penis, usually pretty vigorously, to stimulate it. When girls masturbate, they may touch their breasts, rub their clitoris or vagina. Basically, masturbation involves touching or rubbing yourself in whatever way makes you feel good sexually. There's nothing dangerous about it (as long as it doesn't consume your free time), and it is actually quite normal. For many teenagers, masturbation is a way to enjoy their sexual urges without risking sexual activity or intercourse with another person. Masturbation (just masturbation with yourself) can't cause pregnancy and can't cause sexually transmitted diseases. And if you've ever heard that it will make you grow hair on your palms, make you go blind or that other people can tell you masturbate by looking at you, we hope you know by now that that's not true. Duh.

There's another term called **mutual masturbation**. Think of it as masturbation with someone else. That means that one person will touch the other person sexually and vice versa without having intercourse. Some people call this "outercourse" because it doesn't involve intercourse. It's also called heavy petting or a "hand job." Like masturbation, this isn't dangerous if the "masturbators" are only using their hands. Once it goes beyond a hand job to closer skin-to-skin contact or mouth-to-skin contact, then we're talking about a different topic and increased risks. We'll talk more about this in chapter 9.

Oral Sex

If touching each other sexually involves using your mouth or tongue to stimulate another person's genitals, it's called oral sex. Some people call it "going down" on someone. If a girl puts her mouth over a guy's penis, the scientific word for that is fellatio, but most people refer to it as oral sex or a blow job. Blow? We don't think blowing on the penis is really involved; that's just a term people use. When a guy uses his mouth or tongue on a girl's clitoris or vaginal area, the scientific word for that is cunnilingus. There is no nice way to describe it in everyday language; we prefer to stick with the term oral sex.

Anal Sex

Bet you can guess what this means. It means penis in anus. As you can imagine, the anus has loads of bacteria and is not really built for that, so it can be much more risky and cause infection, as well as be painful. Some girls think that if they have anal sex, they are being "abstinent" and can still be a "virgin." But basically, anal sex is just as intimate as vaginal sex, and as we've discussed, the virginity issue is very questionable.

What Is SEXUAL and What Is ABSTINENCE?

There's a lot of talk out there about abstinence. Lots of federal money and entire educational programs have been designed to promote sexual abstinence until marriage. The problem is, many of these programs don't define sexual abstinence very well, so teens are making up their own definitions.

The word *abstain* means to withhold or "not do" something. Like abstaining from drugs means you don't use them. So what is sexual abstinence? Well, it depends on your definition of SEXUAL. We've spent a lot of time talking about sexual feelings and physical touch that is sexual. Is it sexual to hug someone? French kiss? Touch private body parts through your clothes? Sure. All that stuff creates sexual feelings, so it is a sexual thing. But is that what these programs mean? You can't kiss until you are married? We don't think so, but some people's definitions might mean that.

Whether these recommendations are based on religious teachings or just on common sense, the whole reason for encouraging sexual abstinence for all young people is to prevent unwanted pregnancy, sexually transmitted infections and emotional pain that can come from having sex when you're not ready. That means you should abstain from any activity that can cause these problems.

Let's be more precise just for the record. We hope you know how a pregnancy occurs by now, so obviously sexual abstinence means no penis-in-vagina because that could lead to pregnancy. Also, to prevent infections, sexual abstinence would include abstaining from oral sex, anal sex and very close skin-to-skin contact, particularly of the genital areas. Finally, the emotional pain thing is the most difficult to figure out. It may be impossible to prevent emotional pain if you let yourself have strong feelings for others. We can't help having our feelings and emotions hurt in life. But, if you use your *Girl Power* to keep yourself from doing sexual things you don't feel comfortable doing or don't feel ready to do, you're doing the best you can to protect your emotions related to sexual activity. And believe us, there's a very strong link between our emotions and what we do sexually.

So don't fall into the trap of believing that sexual abstinence means you can do anything sexually except have a penis in the vagina. It's not that easy. Think about it, and make a decision you feel good about.

The **Consequences** of Sex

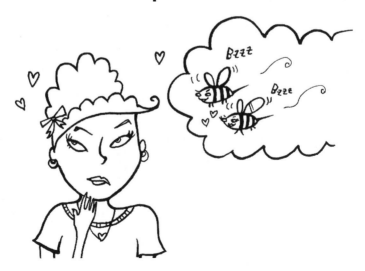

Let us first emphasize that most young teens do not have sexual intercourse, neither vaginal nor anal. These days, teens may be having more oral sex, thinking that it is risk free. Wrong! Any type of sexual contact carries risks, as we'll explain. That means it requires responsible behavior and thinking ahead to avoid those risks.

Obviously, pregnancy is a huge risk that you take if you have sex. There are many effective ways to prevent pregnancy, but nothing except abstinence from sex is 100 percent effective. Most important, pregnancy and childbirth change lives forever—yours, your baby's (obviously!) and your partner's—so it better be something you are prepared to handle if you are going to have sex. Children born to young mothers do not get the same opportunities as children born to adults, who can provide financially and emotionally for a child. Young mothers are also less likely to finish their education, and you can imagine how hard it is to get a good job and provide for your family if you don't have a good education.

Besides getting pregnant from sex, there are infections and diseases that can be passed from one person to another through sexual activities. You've probably heard of some of them. HIV/AIDS is one of the most well known because it kills the people who are infected with it. Other diseases may not be deadly, but they can cause serious problems, such as severe pain, birth defects, infertility (meaning a woman can't get pregnant) and even cancer. You know what's really scary? Every year, one in four teenage girls who have sex will get a sexually transmitted infection. One in four!!! That's a lot! Pretty serious, huh?

Some infections can be treated, but some cannot be treated at all. Some have NO symptoms and can cause infection in the vagina, the uterus or the throat (through oral sex). The biggest problem is that you can never tell for sure whether someone has an infection. Even though a person may get "checked" for sexually transmitted infections, it doesn't mean they don't have ANY infections. That's because there are no reliable and easy tests for some of the most common infections like the human papilloma virus (this causes genital warts and can lead to cervical cancer) and herpes. If someone is checked, it is usually only for gonorrhea and chlamydia (by putting a small cotton swab into the urethra or taking a urine sample) and for HIV, hepatitis and syphilis (by drawing blood). There are lots of other possible infections for which we don't or can't test.

The only 100 percent effective way to avoid infections is not to do the stuff that passes on these infections—and that means NO sexual intercourse, including oral sex.

For people who are having sex, there are ways to help prevent infections and pregnancy. **Condoms,** which are these little balloonlike things that fit over a guy's erect penis before it goes in the vagina (also called a "rubber"), will block the sperm from getting inside the vagina. It will also cover most of the penis, so infection doesn't spread through the skin. Since condoms don't cover all of the skin around the bottom of the penis or the testicles, **they don't completely prevent the diseases that are passed by skin-to-skin contact.** Those infections are the ones that cause things like genital warts, cervical cancer and herpes ulcers. So condoms **can't prevent all infections but they are still very important if you are having sex.**

Why use them if they don't work? They DO work but not 100 percent of the time. For now, if you decide to have sex, condoms are the only thing available that can help reduce the risks of sexually transmitted infections.

Condoms can also help prevent pregnancy, but they are by no means foolproof because they can be used improperly, or they can break or tear. There are other methods of **birth control** that women and men use to prevent pregnancy. Some types of birth control kill sperm in the vagina (spermicide), some block sperm (condoms, diaphragm), and some prevent a woman from ovulating (birth control pills, shots, patches) or prevent an egg from settling into the endometrium (intrauterine device and other hormonal methods like birth control pills). While birth control helps prevent pregnancy, the only 100 percent effective way to avoid pregnancy is to not have sex. Using birth control requires a lot of self-control and planning, and it can be costly. If you are or plan on having sex, you need a birth control plan, and you should talk to your parents, another adult you trust or your doctor. Don't just let sex happen without a plan for protecting yourself from unintended pregnancy and infections.

The take-home message: The only 100 percent effective way to prevent pregnancy and sexually transmitted infections is to avoid sexual intercourse and other sexual activities that put you at risk. But there are plenty of other things you can do to enjoy a romantic relationship. Stay tuned!

Is That **All** There Is to It?

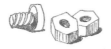

Well, kinda sorta. That's sex in a nutshell, the good and the bad, the nuts and bolts, birds and bees part of it, at least. But as the rest of this book points out, **sex is never just the nuts and bolts.** It has major emotional, physical and relationship effects—many of which are wonderful, provided you are physically and emotionally mature enough to have sex. And it has the most awesome, amazing power in the world: to create a new life! Girls with Girl Power not only **understand the how-to's of sex,** they respect the awesomeness of that tiny little word.

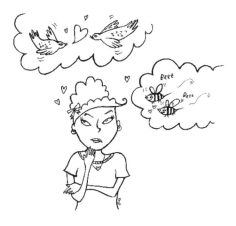

READER/CUSTOMER CARE SURVEY

We care about your opinions! Please take a moment to fill out our online Reader Survey at **http://survey.hcibooks.com.**
As a **"THANK YOU"** you will receive a **VALUABLE INSTANT COUPON** towards future book purchases as well as a **SPECIAL GIFT** available only online! Or, you may mail this card back to us and we will send you a copy of our exciting catalog with your valuable coupon inside.

(PLEASE PRINT IN ALL CAPS)

First Name		MI.	Last Name
Address			City
State	Zip		Email:

1. Gender
- ❑ Female   ❑ Male

2. Age
- ❑ 8 or younger
- ❑ 9-12   ❑ 13-16
- ❑ 17-20   ❑ 21-30
- ❑ 31+

3. Did you receive this book as a gift?
- ❑ Yes   ❑ No

4. How did you find out about the book
- ❑ Friend
- ❑ School
- ❑ Parent

- ❑ Online
- ❑ Store Display
- ❑ Teen Magazine
- ❑ Interview/Review

5. Where do you usually buy books
(please choose one)
- ❑ Bookstore
- ❑ Online
- ❑ Book Club/Mail Order
- ❑ Price Club (Sam's Club, Costco's, etc.)
- ❑ Retail Store (Target, Wal-Mart, etc.)

6. What magazines do you like to read *(please choose one)*
- ❑ Teen People
- ❑ Seventeen
- ❑ YM
- ❑ Cosmo Girl
- ❑ Rolling Stone
- ❑ Teen Ink
- ❑ Christian Magazines
- ❑ Series Books (Chicken Soup, Fearless, etc.)

8. What attracts you most to a book
(please choose one)
- ❑ Title
- ❑ Cover Design
- ❑ Author
- ❑ Content

7. What books do you like to read *(please choose one)*
- ❑ Fiction
- ❑ Self-help
- ❑ Reality Stories/Memoirs
- ❑ Sports

TAPE IN MIDDLE; DO NOT STAPLE

BUSINESS REPLY MAIL
FIRST-CLASS MAIL PERMIT NO 45 DEERFIELD BEACH, FL

POSTAGE WILL BE PAID BY ADDRESSEE

HCI Teens
3201 SW 15th Street
Deerfield Beach FL 33442-9875

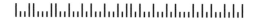

FOLD HERE

Comments

PART THREE

There's **More** to Sex!

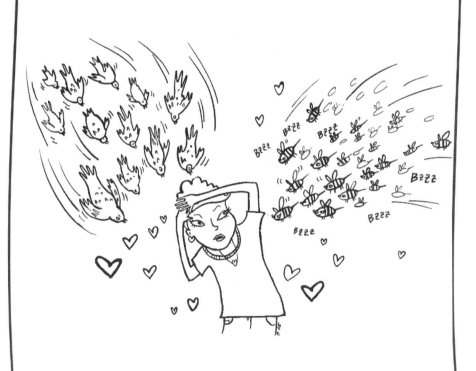

9

Sexuality: Good News, Bad News

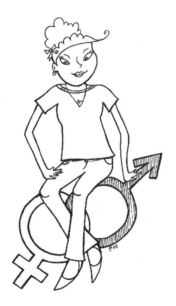

So girls, here's the scoop: Despite all the rumors and whispers, it's not all about sex! And better yet, **you don't have to "do it" to be sexual or sexy.** While we are rumor bashing, we also want to remind you one more time that most young teens do NOT have sexual intercourse. That doesn't mean they aren't sexual.

All people are sexual whether or not they have sex. How can that be? It has to do with this bigger thing called sexuality.

Feeling Sexy?

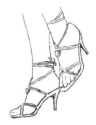

By now, you know that your body and your brain are going through some major changes. That means you are having some thoughts and feelings that are new to you, and whether you want to admit it or not, some of these feelings are sexual. It's another one of those things that happens to you. You can't help it, so don't freak out when it happens. **It's normal!** You are supposed to be having sexual feelings. It's what you do with those feelings and urges that matters!!!

What types of sexual feelings do young teens have? Mostly you're probably very curious. You want to know more:

- About your body
- About other girls' or boys' bodies
- About sex

You may want to look at pictures or read about sex. You may be attracted to boys or girls in a different way than just friendship. You may feel like you want to hang out with your crush all the time, to hold hands or to kiss.

So What **Is** It?

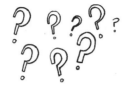

Sexuality includes a lot of important stuff: like how comfortable you are with your own **body** and how you enjoy it; like **intimacy**, which is physical and emotional closeness with another person; like **sexual iden-tity** which deals with the way you feel about being female and how it affects you sexually; like the **consequences** of sex and how prepared you are to deal with all of them; like the use of sex to have **power or con-trol** over other people.

Sexuality is about more than an action or "doing it," **it's about values, beliefs, emotions and attitudes.** That's a lot to cover, so let's break it down.

You Are Sexual
Whether You **Like It or Not**

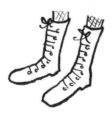

As we've said over and over: Maturing sexually is a major part of being a teenager. **It's a big task.** One of the most important things for you to do during this process of maturing is to notice and appreciate the amaz-ing changes that your body is making.

Lots of girls don't feel good about their bodies. They may buy into all the "beautiful" people advertisements in magazines or on TV that make us think that our bodies should look like Barbie. Do you know how many girls actually have a body like the ones you see in the ads? Less than 1 percent . . . and many of those girls and women are unhealthy. We'll talk more about the media and how it affects us in chapter 10.

Girls also might have confusing feelings about their body because all these changes are happening so fast and they have NO control over them. **Like to be in control?** We do! Well, by eating healthy and getting some type of exercise every day, you can have a little more control about how well your body works. Remember, how your body works is so much more important than how it looks.

Horny?!

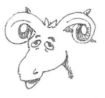

Now, the way your body works sexually involves more than periods and vaginas and clitorises. That's just the "plumbing." What really drives us sexually is our feeling of desire—desire to be close to someone, desire to touch and be touched, desire to explore sexual feelings. Another word for desire is *libido,* but when a person has sexual urges, most teens call that feeling "horny."

Interestingly, **nobody ever seems interested in talking to teens about their sexual desire.** Everyone just seems to expect you to "just say

no." Well, feelings are one of those things that just happen to you; you can't help it. As early as the start of puberty, sexual desire is a feeling that just happens to pop up from time to time.

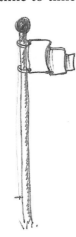

Speaking of popping up . . . boys have an advantage here. When they have sexual desire or sexual thoughts, they get an erection. It's like a flag going up to say, "Hey dude, you're noticing something sexual, and I'm here to point that out!" Is there a similar flag for girls? We don't get such an obvious "pop up" (thank goodness!). For girls, the signal is more subtle and brainy—kind of like we are anyway, right?

When girls have sexual feelings, the major signal comes through our thoughts—stuff like, "I want to hold your hand," or "I want to think about marrying you," or "I want to kiss you," or maybe, "I want to ride a horse on the beach with you." Sexual thoughts are never harmful, but acting upon them is where the risks can occur. **So go ahead, enjoy your thoughts,** picture yourself kissing your favorite movie star, think about marrying your crush, daydream about your true love all you want. It's normal.

Skin Hunger

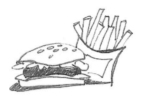

Another part of desire that you may also be noticing is a physical thing that can be called "skin hunger." Teen girls and boys are very huggy and touchy sometimes. Your parents probably satisfied your skin hunger when you were a child—all that cuddling and loving and sitting on their laps. Now that you are spending less time with parents and more time with friends, it's normal to look to your friends for that special touch. It's also normal to sometimes want to be touched or hugged by your boyfriend or crush.

As you notice skin hunger, you may also notice a **physical feeling in your genital area.** This is a reflex that is part of sexual desire, and it signals that your brain is starting to grow in the romance department. Some girls and women describe the genital feelings of desire as fullness, warmth, tingling or a twinge. Along with that sensation, another reflex makes the vagina release fluids that make it feel wet. Some girls have no clue this happens unless they touch the vaginal area and feel it. Other girls have enough lubrication to make their underwear get wet. It's not the same "wetness" that happens with normal vaginal discharge, but it, too, is normal with sexual desire.

Remember, guys get lots and lots of erections as teens, and girls also have many sexual thoughts and feelings. But just because a boy gets an erection or a girl has sexual feelings doesn't mean they have to have sex.

Neither boys nor girls NEED to have sex, and in fact, most don't. Instead, you need to learn to recognize and appreciate your sexual arousal in ways other than intercourse. There are lots of ways to enjoy these sexual feelings without having sex. Sometimes, you can just sit back and enjoy the feeling and **know that your body is working like it's meant to.**

Solo Sex Revisited

Some teens masturbate when these sexual urges are strong. That can let them release some sexual urges in a safe way and get on with other things. It's weird to talk about masturbation and even weirder to think about whether it's okay or not. Let us assure you that most people masturbate at some point in their lives, but few will admit it. Keep in mind, **it's not a popular dinner conversation, it's not a group activity, and it shouldn't consume your free time,** but it is both safe and normal.

Should you ask your parents if it's okay to masturbate? That's up to you. A lot of parents will get totally freaked out if you ask, even though they may think it's fine. That's because they don't want to know you are having sexual feelings. Kind of like the way you don't want to believe that your parents "do it." But if parents consider the options—(1) you relieve your own sexual urges versus (2) you look for someone else to relieve them for you—most parents would agree: help yourself! But **pleeeeze keep it private!** If you need to relieve sexual urges, we would bet that you can learn to make yourself feel better sexually than any awkward teenage boy can try to make you feel. And remember, just because you have sexual urges doesn't mean you *need* to do anything at all!

Warm **Fuzzies**

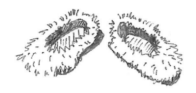

Being intimate is the heart and soul of a mature relationship. **Intimacy is a two-way street;** it means getting close with someone emotionally and physically in a very comfortable way and having that feeling returned to you. It's hard to talk about with young teens, because it's not a big part of your sexual development until you are older. (It has to do with all the stuff about how your brain is growing and developing. . . .) We'll spare you the details right now, but you need to gain some independence and self-respect and get some experience under your belt before you'll understand true intimacy.

Intimacy doesn't always mean boyfriend-girlfriend or husband-wife stuff. You can also be intimate with your best buds. This means:

- Sharing secrets
- Accepting flaws
- Knowing how to forgive
- Getting to know your friends' likes and dislikes
- Trusting

The list goes on and on, and it's all good. Does this all sound familiar?

It's just like we talked about in the chapter on "friends who rock."

For now, developing intimate friendships, learning to be a good friend, and finding those friends who rock is what you will build on as you get older and develop intimate romantic relationships. Remember, **emotional intimacy should always come before physical intimacy.** That means learning how to be intimate with feelings should come before you try to learn how to be intimate with your body.

Being intimate doesn't come easily, and it can be risky. What do we mean by risky? Well, let's say you tell a friend a secret about a very embarrassing moment for you, but you realize that if she tells everyone that secret, you would feel humiliated. By telling your secret to a friend, you risk everyone else finding out something you don't want anyone else to know. Part of what you will learn as a young teen is who you can trust and become intimate with. It's more important for you right now to learn to be a good friend and find good friends. This should all happen before you head off on any romantic journey.

What Is **Girly**?

What does it mean to be a girl? Does it mean you have to wear dresses, get your ears pierced and fantasize about boys? Does it mean you have to want to have babies? Does it mean you can't be a firefighter or a professional athlete? Heck no! Being a girl only means you were born with certain genes and parts, and **all the rest is up to you.** Sometimes that's not the message we hear or how we feel, though. We get ideas from our families, from the media, from our peers and all of society about how girls are "supposed" to be. But a girl with Girl Power **can't be forced into a girly thing that doesn't feel right for her.**

What if you like to wear camo pants and a baseball hat? What if a guy enjoys ballet? What if you enjoy baseball over gymnastics? What if you like short hair? What if you aren't interested in kissing boys? That's cool. It's about expressing your personal preferences, which is what teens on the road toward independence and adulthood are supposed to be doing. Some people, though, might not be comfortable with your individuality and might call you names. Teens, as we're sure you know, can be **cruel with their name calling,** and one of the names you'll hear for guys who do things that are considered more "girly" is "faggot" or "homo." Girls who like things that are more popular with boys might be called "dykes" or "lesbians." These words are hurtful. Doing things differently or having certain interests doesn't mean anything about a person's sexual orientation.

Straight **or** Gay

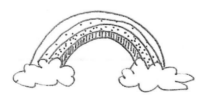

So what IS sexual orientation? First of all, sexual orientation is not at all about how you look. It may not even be about whom you have kissed. It is really about who you are attracted to in a romantic way. If a male is emotionally and physically attracted in a mature romantic way to another male, then he is homosexual. Same goes for females attracted to females—they are homosexual. The word *homosexual* means the same thing as the word *gay*. Homosexual women are also called *lesbians*. **Some people use hurtful words** when talking about gay people, but the most respectful words to use are *gay* and *lesbian*.

There are also some people who are sexually attracted to both males and females. They are called *bisexual*. If a male is attracted to females or a female is attracted to males, they are *heterosexual*. Ninety percent of the people in the world are heterosexual.

But love is love. We can't always help who we fall in love with. The world is filled with enough hatred and violence. We should never hate people for loving others—even if it means they are gay.

Am I Gay?

Believe it or not, this question is common and normal, and most young teens wonder about it at some point. Remember, you are trying to figure out who you are sexually, so you may think about all the possibilities. While all this sex stuff is going on in your body and brain, you may find yourself having sexual thoughts about another girl or woman. You will certainly look at other girls when they are undressing in the gym or at a sleepover. You might have even touched another girl in a private or sexual way. **Don't freak out.** At your age, this happens sometimes and doesn't mean anything yet about your sexual orientation. In fact, around age twelve or thirteen, about one in four girls can't say for sure whether they think they are gay or not. But by age eighteen, only one in twenty girls doesn't know for sure. That means that during adolescence, most girls figure out and feel comfortable about their sexual orientation. It can be a tough and confusing thing to think you are gay during your teen years. It is really important to **find someone you can talk to openly.** If you don't think your parents are the ones, look to a school counselor, doctor, a friend's parent or other trusted adult.

There is a lot of controversy about whether people choose to be homosexual or whether they are born that way. We aren't here to answer that question, but it is very important to realize that people are people, and their sexual orientation means nothing about their value as humans. **Being gay is not easy** in our society because of teasing and discrimination. We should treat each other with **respect and tolerance,** which is what girls with Girl Power do.

Sex and **Power**: It Can Be Good, It Can Be Bad

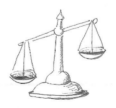

Sexuality is powerful. Advertising companies have used the power of sexual images for many years because it works. Sex sells. They might show a photo of a big-breasted woman on a motorcycle to sell a pair of jeans, but what do her breasts have to do with the jeans? They may show a sexy pair of legs with a sports drink next to them to sell that drink. What do the legs have to do with the sports drink? Absolutely nothing, nada, zippo. But the image of something sexy always seems to get attention. It's powerful.

We bet some of your classmates have figured this out, too. A special glance, an innocent touch or a certain comment might actually send a message that says, "Hey, look at me, I'm kind of cute, and I'm looking at you . . . yeah you." That, we're sure you know, is called *flirting*. **Flirting can be innocent and fun.** It's a way that girls and guys let each other know there's an interest brewing. On the other hand, **flirting can become not so good** if it turns into excessive teasing or manipulating behavior.

Sexual **Harassment**

Sometimes flirting goes too far and may make you feel uncomfortable. For instance, a cute guy in your class starts staring at you, and every time you look at him, he winks. Flattered? Maybe. Let's say he then starts following you in the halls and whispers comments about how nice your breasts look to him. How does that make you feel? Probably **very uncomfortable.** This is a form of sexual harassment.

How about if you're walking through a crowded hallway at school, and someone pinches or fondles your butt. Some girls might think this attention is cool, but unwanted attention of that kind is also a form of sexual harassment.

The more common examples of sexual harassment are when someone uses sexual language, talks about sex, or uses touch or body language in a way that makes you feel uncomfortable, embarrassed or threatened. Another type of sexual harassment is when someone asks you to look at photos of naked people or sexual acts (also called **pornography**). They can even send them to you through the Internet when you don't even want to look at that stuff. Why would someone do this? It's a power trip. They are using words, actions or physical contact to feel more powerful than you. Remember, **sexual harassment is not only wrong, it is illegal.** If you feel like someone is harassing you, it's time to talk to that good old trusted adult.

When Sex Is a **Crime**

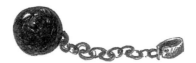

Unfortunately, there are people in this world who use the power of sex in very bad ways. If an adult forces you or talks you into doing something sexual that you don't want to do, it's called **sexual abuse**. If they take photographs of you naked or doing sexual things, it's pornography, and that is sexual abuse as well. It's a way they take advantage of children or teens for their own pleasure or entertainment—sometimes just for the power trip of it. **Sexual abusers are not just spooky-looking men, they can be anybody, even adults who supervise kids and seem to like them.** Sometimes sexual abuse occurs within families (this is called **incest**). How can this happen? Abusers will often earn the trust of the child by buying gifts or providing treats, but then they expect the child to keep secrets about what's happening in private. They may threaten to stop the gifts or even threaten to withdraw love if the child tells anyone. Sometimes they threaten to hurt someone the child loves if the child tells anyone. And even if the child does tell, people may have a hard time believing them. The child might even be afraid that no one will believe them.

No matter who it is—a parent, a coach, a friend of the family, a step-parent, a neighbor—anyone who does this is a criminal, because **sexual abuse is illegal,** and the abusers are way sick in the head. Unfortunately, it happens more than you would ever imagine. If this has ever happened to you or anyone you know, your first step is to **tell an adult** who will listen and help. If you aren't sure who you can tell, a good resource is a school counselor.

Rape

Rape (also called *sexual assault*) is when someone is forced into sexual activity. Most of the time, girls are raped by boys or men. If a male forces his penis, finger, tongue or other object into a female's vagina, anus or mouth, it is rape. This is a violent crime, and there is **no excuse for it.** It has very little to do with sex but a lot to do with power. Even though it seems like a sexual kind of thing, rapists do not rape for sexual feelings. Instead, **rapists rape for power and control.**

Unfortunately, when many girls and women are raped, they do not tell anyone or report it to the police because they feel embarrassed or ashamed. No matter how a girl acts or dresses, **nothing makes it okay for someone to rape her.** Some girls even think they might be partly to blame for it happening, and many girls think they are "ruined" or have "lost their virginity" to a rapist. That's why rape can confuse girls and make them feel bad about themselves. If you are raped, you aren't ruined, because it is something that happened *to* you. You didn't have a choice in it, and most girls do whatever it takes just to survive the experience. What *you* do have a choice about is taking care of yourself and getting medical attention so you can heal from it, both physically and emotionally.

Most girls think that rapes happen only in dark alleys or when girls hitchhike. The awful truth is that **most girls who are raped are raped by someone they know** or have met recently. Most rapes also happen in someone's home (or apartment or dorm) or another familiar place.

Unfortunately, most rapes happen to teenage girls, and one of the most common types of rape is called **date rape.** Like it sounds, this happens when a girl is out with a guy she may like, and he forces her to have sex with him. Sometimes the force is real physical force, but sometimes it is by **talking her into it** when she doesn't really want to. Sometimes she says no, but he doesn't listen, and many times, **drugs or alcohol** are involved. This is another good reason to "just say no" to drugs and alcohol. Even in date rape or drug-related rape, girls still need to get medical attention afterward to help prevent infections and pregnancy and to make sure there are no injuries. The sooner a girl gets medical attention, the better for preventing infections and pregnancy as well as for making sure the victim is okay. If this ever happens to you or someone you know, it is also important to get help to heal emotionally. Going to an emergency room or your doctor is important for getting this type of help.

Again, rape is a crime. It needs to be reported to the police or an adult who can help, and **immediate medical attention is very important.** Guys who rape once often do it again and again to other girls. By reporting the crime, you can help prevent that. It's a horrible shame that rape happens, but there's no reason for the victim to feel ashamed. Tell all your girlfriends that the most important thing is to get help.

No Means No!

Even if you want to mess around and you say it's okay, sometimes sex can still be a crime. A crime? Yep. Let's look at a real-life story:

A 14-year-old girl and her boyfriend are kissing and move into heavy petting. She starts to feel uneasy with their actions and asks her boyfriend to stop. He is so sexually excited that he doesn't listen and doesn't stop. They end up having sex.

There is a huge problem here. When two people are involved in sexual behaviors, they both have to agree to what they are doing. This is called **consent,** and it matters a ton! In fact, if someone does not give consent to sex, it is rape. The important thing about consent is that it should be "active," meaning you both actually agree to sex or sexual touching by saying yes. "Passive" consent doesn't count, because that's when you don't say anything, so he *assumes* you are okay going along with it. You can't just assume what others want when it comes to something as personal as sex. So again, sex without consent is rape. As you already know, rape is a crime that is punished by law and can mean prison.

What about the situation above where this is her boyfriend and she was okay with the petting, but not with going all the way? She wouldn't want to get her boyfriend in trouble, but what he did is absolutely wrong.

Remember, **rape is a power issue, not a sex issue.** Guys who don't stop when asked aren't interested in the girl or her feelings. They are only interested in their own power over her. Any guy can stop, even in the middle of sex, and it won't hurt him in any way . . . so there's no excuse. No means NO! Stop means STOP! **Be clear about what you want and don't want.**

What about times when you don't say no but don't want to go further? You can try body language, like turning away, pulling his hand away, closing your legs together. But guys are NOT good at understanding body language, especially in the heat of the moment. So you have to find your voice, no matter how hard, and utter the words, "STOP . . . I don't want to do this." A true love will understand and respect your feelings. A true love will wait until the time is right for both of you.

What Does the **Law** Have to Do With Me and My Sex Life?!

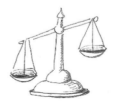

Another big issue with consent is that you have to be ABLE to GIVE consent. That means you have to be **old enough** and you have to have a clear mind. Old enough? Yes. States have laws that say when a teen is old enough to "consent" to having sex. The age is different among different states, but in general, it ranges from 14 to 17 years of age.

There are reasons for these laws. When you are a young teen, even though you are smart and mature for your age, you still are not ready to handle all of the things that go along with having sex. **This is so important that every state has this kind of law.** That means that if a guy tries to have sex with a girl who is younger than the age of consent, it is illegal. Even if the girl says yes, it doesn't matter because the state says she isn't old enough to give permission. It would be like you trying to sign your own report card or permission slip. It's not allowed, and the rules are very clear.

Finally and importantly, people who are under the influence of alcohol or drugs are not ABLE to give consent. That means that **if a girl is drunk,** and a guy has sex with her, it is illegal because she can't give consent. This is also rape and punishable by law.

Scary, huh? Unfortunately, this is how a lot of girls end up having sex when they don't mean to. Remember how we said that **you have the power to make choices that help you stick to your boundaries—**choices like not getting drunk or high, not being alone with a guy you're not sure you can trust, or not going so far that it's hard to stop before you have sex? Well, even if you make a poor decision, get drunk and end up in a bad situation, you do not deserve to be raped! If you are not able to give consent to sex, if you say NO or if you are too young to give consent, the sex is a crime. And the guy is wrong and can be punished by the law!

If anything like this happens to you, speak up! Get help! Tell your parents, a teacher at school, a girlfriend's mom—find someone who can help you. It will be tough. You may even feel like it was your fault if you were where you shouldn't have been, doing things you shouldn't have been doing or with people you shouldn't have been with. **Find your courage!** It is not your fault, and a guy who forces sex on you, no matter what the circumstances, is a criminal.

Healthy Sexuality

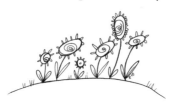

We know that some of this stuff about sexuality and power sounds scary, and it is. The ways that people can abuse sex for power and for harm are really rotten. But remember, there is good power, too. There's Girl Power. **Learning to understand and use your sexuality in healthy ways is a big part of Girl Power;** it can help you be in control and keep you healthy and safe.

There is great power that comes from knowledge and making good choices about your body and what it can do. Your body is the tool you will use to enjoy your sexuality all your life, so it is important that you take good care of it and treat it with respect. Here's how you develop the Girl Power that comes with healthy sexuality:

- You understand and **accept the changes** happening in your body.
- You do what you can to keep your body **healthy.**
- You notice that you have **sexual feelings.**
- You learn to appreciate your sexual feelings, but you act on them in a **safe and responsible way.**

- You feel comfortable **discussing sexual issues** with your parents or another trusted adult.
- You are **respectful** of other people's sexual identities and choices but **stand up for your own values.**
- You rely on your friends to help you learn about **trust** and **being intimate** with feelings.
- You understand that some people use **sex for power.**
- You look forward to a fulfilling sexual experience in a relationship that is **meaningful and responsible;** for most people, that means in a mature, committed adult relationship or marriage.

That's what Girl Power and *Girlology* is all about. So feel good about your sexuality! It's a big part of who you are and who we hope you'll become—a healthy, strong, smart young woman who's got it going on, body, mind and soul!

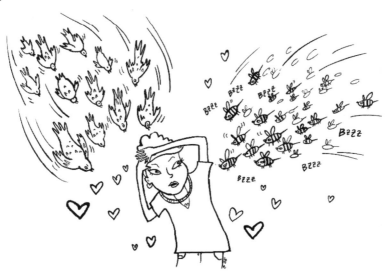

10

Mixed Messages

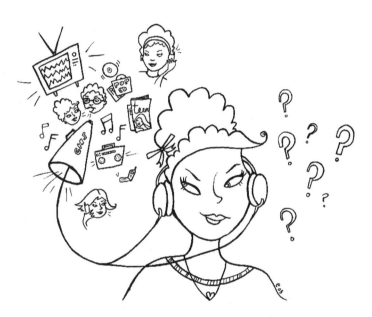

Sex is a hot topic. Just check out the cover of *Seventeen* magazine, the posters in your health class, TV shows, religious youth group programs and the rows of books on sexuality in Barnes & Noble. **Everybody's got something to say about sex.**

With all these different people weighing in on sex, it can be a confusing topic. So confusing that we can't even agree on what to call it! In science we call it "reproduction." Your parents might call it "making love." Friends can call it "sleeping" with a boy. It's called sex, sexual intercourse, as well as lots of not-so-proper names.

Why do we have so many names for it? And why are some of the names "nice" and some aren't nice at all? The reason is simple. Different people have lots of different ideas about sex. Some think it's loving affection between husband and wife. Others think it's just a fun way to relieve yourself when you feel sexually aroused or "horny." Some people say sex is mainly for making babies. Other people do it for the sheer thrill and excitement. What a variety of ideas! **What a bag of mixed messages!**

With all these mixed messages, how do we decide what's right for us? Where do we get the information that helps us decide? Parents? Television? Church? Movies? Boyfriends? Teachers? Friends? Magazines? Internet?

Whom do you listen to? How do you decide which messages are important and which are not so important? It's hard! If you are like a lot of girls, you want to:

- Fit in with your **friends**
- Be liked by **boys**
- Be trusted by your **parents**
- Know about the **latest trends**

Parents, girlfriends, boyfriends and the media can have different ideas about how your friends, boys, parental trust and trends fit in with your new sexual self. If you are paying attention to all these messages, here's what you might hear:

From Parents

I'm glad you asked me.

What?! Why are you interested in sex? Are you
already doing it?

Wait until you're married.

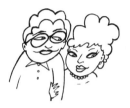

Use birth control.

Sex is a gift you save for your husband.

Sex is dirty.

Sex is not healthy for teenagers.

Sex is for adults only.

Sex is wonderful if you are in the right relationship.

Sex is dangerous.

Sex is intimate and emotional.

Sex is a gift from God.

From Girlfriends

I want to have sex now.

I want to wait until I'm married
to have sex.

Sex is gross.

I can't believe you haven't had sex yet!

Sex is disappointing.

Sex is fun.

Sex is all about the guys.

Sex is something that everyone is doing.

Sex is scary.

You need to use a condom.

You only need to have sex if you want a baby.

Boys only like you if you have sex.

My boyfriend wanted to do it, so I did.

My boyfriend wants to wait. Is that weird?

Once you start having sex, it's really hard to stop.

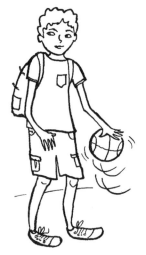

From Boyfriends

Guys have to have it to release tension.

Let's wait until we are both ready to do sexual things.

Your sense of humor is what I love best about you.

It gets me hot when you wear that micro-mini with the baby T.

Everybody is doing it.

We'll just stop at second base.

From Magazines, TV and Movies

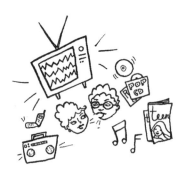

Sex is no big deal.

Sex is exciting.

Sex feels good.

You will be happy if you have sex.

Sex is always romantic and passionate.

You need big boobs to be sexy.

You need a skinny body to be sexy.

You need tight jeans to be attractive to guys.

You need a lot of makeup and perfect skin to have sex appeal.

Everybody has sex with every boyfriend they ever have.

You don't even need to have a husband or a boyfriend to have sex! Just do it for fun!

What Else Have You Heard?

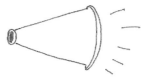

There's a lot of contradiction here, isn't there? They can't all be right, so who is?

Decision time! *You* have to decide what is right. And "right" here doesn't mean the same thing it does on a test. No way. Right means what is healthy for your body, your emotions and your relationships—now and in the future. Your job is to check out all the messages you get and then decide what your own opinion is. Decide what is healthy for you.

We've said it before, but it's important enough to say again: Some of the people telling you about sex are interested in what's best for *you*. They are usually people in relationships with you, people you know well and who care about you when it comes to things other than sex. Others are interested in what's best for *them*. They usually want to sell you something or get their own way.

So how do you respond to these ideas and pressures? We've just reviewed the messages themselves, now let's talk about why they are so mixed up.

Oh No, "**The** Talk"

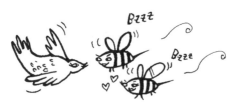

Lots of **parents feel really awkward** talking about sex. Maybe it's because their parents didn't talk with them. Or maybe they just can't picture their baby girl as a sexual being. Some parents regret sexual choices they made as teens and are afraid to tell you about it.

It's hard for parents to imagine you as even thinking about sexual things. But their little girl is growing up (sniff, sniff), and they see you changing a lot. You probably choose clothes and wear makeup to make yourself attractive to guys. You go to "boy-girl parties" where you hang out and maybe even flirt and dance with guys. You might even start to date. **Cut your parents some slack!** This isn't exactly easy on them either!

Parents handle the sex talk in lots of different ways. Do any of these sound familiar?

1. "Read this book." Some parents try to ignore the topic completely and just hand over a book like this one. As useful as this book is, it can't replace honest conversation. If your parents **hand you a book and then run in** the opposite direction, chase them down and ask questions! Be brave and start the sex conversation yourself!

2. "You'll get pregnant, never finish high school and end up working at McDonald's your entire life if you have sex." **Yikes! Scare tactics! Guilt!** That pregnant/school dropout/McDonald's thing

certainly can happen, but your sexuality involves a lot more than just having sexual intercourse. It can be holding hands, kissing, touching, sharing secrets, emotional closeness and friendship. But sometimes parents are so afraid you will make a big mistake with sex that they are afraid to let you open the door on your sexuality in any way, shape or form. *You'll* have to open that door. Respect their privacy, but ask them what choices they made as teens that they are happy with now, twenty or thirty years later. Which ones are they unhappy about? If they don't want to talk about their personal experiences, respect their privacy. Maybe they would rather tell you stories about some of their friends' experiences when they were teens.

3. "I'm so glad you asked me. I've been wanting to talk to you about sex, but I wasn't sure you were interested yet." Some parents have no trouble discussing it at all. They are **open and honest.** They admit their fears and wishes for you as you develop sexually. They explore what a healthy relationship looks like with you and help you identify peer pressure. They give you reasons for wanting you to handle sex a certain way, and they help you decide based on your family's values.

Different parents can give you different messages about sex, but there is one thing you can be pretty certain of. They want what is best for you. Their opinion is one you can respect, **even if they trip all over themselves telling it to you.**

The Talk among **Teens**

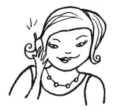

Your friends and your boyfriend are right in the thick of this whole sexual development thing with you. Girlfriends are deciding to hold hands with a guy on Monday, to kiss a guy on Thursday, and then changing their minds again. They are experimenting with clothing and makeup styles that are hot and sexy. In doing that, some are finding out that what they wear can send the wrong message about the type of person they are. They are also figuring out the difference between guy friends, boyfriends and crushes. And why do guy friends turn into crushes so easily these days?

Boyfriends are teens just like you—**figuring this sex thing out as they go along.** Some can be great friends as well as boyfriends. Those are the ones who talk to you about sexual things and respect your wishes. They don't pressure you to do things you don't want to do, and you don't pressure them either. Those are the boyfriends who have what's best for you in mind.

And just like some girlfriends, some guys don't have what's best for you in mind. They are easy to pick out. They are the ones who have *their* best interests in mind—the guys who cause your girlfriends to say, "Sex is all about the boy." They may tell you their bodies *need* sex, or you'll do it if you *love* them, or you're just a prude because *everyone* is doing it. **Wrong, wrong and wrong again!**

Some friends will seem really confident and have tons of information about sex stuff you've never even heard of. But they are not experts. Beware of the information you get from other teens about sex. Lots of it is not true. We know. We hear it from our patients every day. Have you ever heard any of this before?

- You can't get pregnant the first time you have sex.
- You can't get pregnant if you are on your period.
- You can't get any infections from oral sex.
- Sex is no big deal.
- Everyone is doing it.
- Boys have to have sex to release tension.

Guess what. Every single one of these statements is FALSE. Remember, we know from research that most young teens are not having sex, but **a lot of them like to make you** *think* **they are.** Be careful about believing everything a casual friend says about sex. Especially if she sounds like she is bragging or acting superior. It's probably not true. She's more likely trying to show off than help you decide what is best for you.

Now your closest friends *do* want what is best for you. They don't lie to you on purpose. It's just that they don't have all the information you need. But you can count on them to be honest, and together you can read books, talk to trusted adults and find out the truth about sex!

The Talk in the **Media**

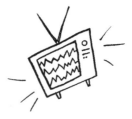

News flash! The media is one group that is *not* worried about what's best for you.

Well, let's take that back for just a minute. There are reporters and shows that provide great factual information that will help you make healthy decisions. And we give them credit. But the media we are talking about are a lot of the advertisers, entertainers and too many shows that are on TV every day. Entire books have been written about how these folks make girls feel bad about themselves and give people wrong impressions about what's normal.

TV shows make you think that sex always occurs suddenly in a moment of passion or hot sexiness. Guess what? Most sex happens in a more planned way where the couple has **thought about it, talked about it and planned for ways to protect themselves** from pregnancy and diseases.

Magazines make you think that sexy women are all ultra skinny, in designer clothes and with perfect skin. Wrong again. Most women are nothing like that. In fact those women in the magazines aren't really like that either! They have professional hair and makeup artists, wardrobe stylists and top-notch photographers whose jobs are to make them look perfect. Plus the photos are airbrushed or manipulated on a computer to cover up blemishes, cellulite and other imperfections before they are printed. **Perfect bodies and skin? We don't think so!**

People get brainwashed into thinking that what they see on TV and in magazines is what's normal. Lots of girls compare themselves with the models and actresses they see and end up feeling bad about their looks or their clothes. If you want to see what's really normal, take a look around your school lunchroom. You'll see girls of all shapes and sizes—short and petite, broad-shouldered and muscular, size 2 and size 16, long hair and short hair, clumsy and graceful. The variety is endless!

Take an **Active** Role!

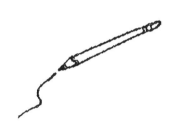

If you are like a lot of teen girls, you like reading magazines and watching TV. But you need to learn how to recognize when advertisers and producers are messing with your head. Fight back. If you see a TV show that is unrealistic—like sex between teens with no mention of birth control, diseases or emotional effects—write to the producer. If you see a magazine article or ad that promotes unrealistic bodies, cut it out and write a letter. Quit buying products that use ads that make girls feel bad about themselves, and send a letter to the company to tell them why. Advertisers want your money. That's the whole reason they make these ads that get attention. Give them the type of attention they deserve—avoid their products and spread the word. Now *that* feels powerful!!

Unmixing the Message

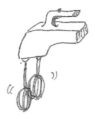

So here you are. Sitting on a pile of mixed and opposite messages about sex. How do you figure it all out?

You can discuss it with the people who want what is best for you. Your close friends, your parents, trusted adults like teachers, doctors, family members and friends' moms.

It works like this. First you get a mixed message. For example, you hear from an "experienced" girl that sex is scary, disappointing and gross. But you know that can't always be true because why then would anyone ever do it? Plus you hear from your mom that it is also wonderful, intimate and a gift to be enjoyed. **You've got to decide which is right!**

Your close friends can help you figure out exactly what things can make sex so yucky—the time, the place, the boy, your age, the relationship, the kind of sexual thing that girl was doing. You can learn from someone else's experience, even if it is bad. If you want nothing less than wonderful when it comes to sexual things, then **promise yourself to stay away from things that make it yucky.** And stick to your promise!

Then go ask your mom what makes sex such a wonderful, intimate gift. Write a list of things that may help make sex a wonderful thing for you some day. **Promise yourself** that you will stick to that list *before* you get caught up in the heat of a passionate moment.

We realize that making a promise to yourself sounds easy, but sticking to it, especially when your peers are pressuring you, is tough. It takes practice. You have to think of some "comebacks" ahead of time and practice using them in different situations. Here are a few examples:

The Pressure	Comebacks
I can't believe you haven't had sex, yet!	I can't believe you have! Oh, then you don't really know me at all. Too bad. I can't believe you think people our age really have sex. They've got you fooled.
If you love him, you'll have sex with him.	If he loves me, he'll wait. I'm worth it. Love's too deep for me right now. I'm just havin' a good time hangin' out with him.
Everyone is doing "it."	I know plenty of people who aren't, so you're wrong. Then I must have a lot more respect for myself than they do. I have a lot of plans for my life, so I'm not going to screw it up by doing something stupid.

You've Got the Power to Decide

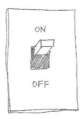

You'll probably find that the mixed messages are *both* true. Sex can be both disappointing and wonderful—depending on when, where, why, how and with whom you do sexual things. It will take some discipline, but the when, where, why, how and with whom are all things you can control. They are all decisions *you* can make.

Different people have lots of different ideas about sex. Some are healthy for you, some are not. But the awesome thing is that *you* have the power to make the ultimate decision about what is healthy and right for you. **Feels nice to be in charge, doesn't it?**

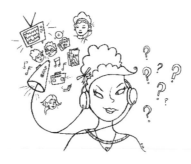

11

Crush or True Love?

So your body is doing strange things, your parents are impossible to figure out, your girlfriends are unpredictable . . . and then there's all this boy craziness!! It's a good thing we're working on Girl Power, because these teen times can seem crazy, especially when you topple head-over-heels for that cute guy in your social studies class. As if there wasn't already enough to worry about, now you're stuck wondering how he really feels about you, or if he's the ONE, or if you'll ever feel okay again after having your heart splintered into a million pieces.

One of the most exciting, wonderful, amazing and absolutely overwhelming parts of being a teenage girl is that **teenage girls (and boys) fall in love.** Or do they? Is it love when you can't sleep at night because you're thinking about seeing HIM at the game tomorrow? Is it love when your heart races at the sight of his number popping up on caller ID? Is it love when you want to drive by his house a thousand times a day just to see if he's home? Is it love that makes you want to be with him, only him and nobody else?

It's *something* all right. Something powerful and fun and very real, but (we hate to break it to you) it's probably not true love.

Did you notice anything about all those things that make you feel "in love"? They are all about excitement. You feel tingly; your heart races; you anticipate seeing him or even knowing where he is. They are great while they last, but feelings of excitement can come and go.

True love is more than just feelings of excitement. Feelings of excitement will definitely be there, but you will also feel at peace around

 him and want to protect him, to build him up so other people will think he's as great as you do and to help him make his goals and dreams come true. And since none of us is perfect (are you surprised?!), true love also makes you want to overlook his weaknesses or those little, unimportant things he does that get on your nerves.

Sound like more than you bargained for? Maybe he does have a killer smile and great sense of humor, but does all this stuff about protecting, building up, fulfilling dreams and overlooking totally annoying habits

seem a little too deep? That's the cool thing about being a teenager! You don't have to commit yourself to a guy in a true-love kind of way yet. You get to practice at it for years before you commit to true love!

Be prepared, because those "in love" feelings of excitement come on fast and strong. So fast and strong that a lot of teens believe they are in love after one or two weeks. Guess what? **True love takes a long time, even years, to grow and strengthen.** What most teens feel (and it is definitely a BEGINNING for love) is a strong attraction, or lust or a crush. Sometimes it's a REALLY strong attraction, and it can be confusing.

It's a **Wild** Ride!

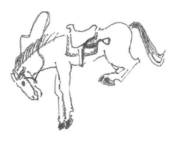

Having a crush is a great feeling. It's exciting, and it makes you happy and all tingly inside. But the whole reason it's called "falling" in love, or being "head over heels" about someone, is because **it throws you off balance.** Crushes have a way of doing just that, "crushing" all your more sensible emotions and other interests. They can take you on a wild, thrilling and often confusing ride of emotions!

Ever have that feeling of being totally consumed by someone? Like your brain simply cannot think about anything else? You're taking a history test and all you can think about is, "I wonder if he brought his lunch or is buying it today. Should I hang out in the lunch line and hope to see him, or maybe he'll be outside at the picnic tables?" You and your girlfriends are planning to see a new movie this weekend, and you're thinking, "Well, he said that movie sounded good. I wonder if he's going to see it this weekend, too. Would he go Friday or Saturday night? At

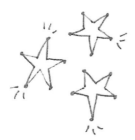

7:00 or 9:00? Maybe I can get someone to call and find out. . . ."

If any of this sounds like you, **you're crushin' . . . big time!**

You can become totally absorbed by your feelings, maybe even obsessed about some-one. You might try to arrange your plans so you see him more often. You might feel jealous if your crush spends time with other people. And you'll definitely feel like you want to please your crush by dressing to impress him, giving him special attention, complimenting him and find-ing things he is interested in to talk about. Flirting comes naturally when you're around a crush! And if he notices you, wow! You feel great!

And if your crush becomes your boyfriend, you may want to please him in other ways, too—perhaps sexually. Part of your attraction probably involves strong sexual urges on your part. But there is a big difference between flirting (which may or may not include holding hands, kissing and making out or exploring some of your body's feelings of attraction) and becoming sexually involved with a crush or a first boyfriend.

What's the Rush?

Just think, if you become intimate or sexually involved with someone early in a relationship, what do you have to look forward to? In this relationship and in future relationships? Too often, teens think that having sex or being involved sexually will make their relationship grow and deepen their commitment to each other. After years of seeing patients and hearing their stories, we can tell you that this definitely is *not* the way it works.

If you want to keep your body, emotions and relationship healthy, a deep commitment and long-lasting relationship should come before sexual involvement and sexual intercourse. Most religions teach that marriage should come before sexual intercourse. There are good reasons for those teachings. When you rush into sexual activity too early, the sex becomes the focus or center of the relationship. Sex is the only thing you do together. Sex is the only thing that's important in the relationship anymore. **If it's too early, you'll feel unfulfilled,** and sex won't seem like such a great thing. Pay attention to those feelings if you have them. They are telling you that you aren't ready.

Once you've "gone all the way," the relationship can lose a lot of the mystery and excitement. There can also be a loss of trust and respect (for

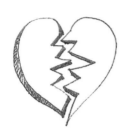

yourself or your partner). There will also be a lot more stress in the relationship because of the responsibilities that go along with being sexually involved. When sex happens too early, the relationship often *ends* shortly after sex *starts* because it didn't have a strong foundation to begin with.

And that can break your heart. Because no matter what movies, TV or other teens might tell you, sex is special, and it is a very big deal. When you give it away to (or have it taken away by) someone who doesn't respect it and you . . . well, that just plain hurts.

If this has already happened to you, if you have already had your heart broken by rushing too quickly into sex, you don't have to keep feeling the hurt over and over again! You can take charge and choose to set limits for physical involvement with your next boyfriend. Your mistake doesn't make you any less lovable or special. If you learn from your mistake, it will even make you wiser. Then the next time you'll be thinking about building a strong foundation for true love, not just giving in to the exciting feelings of a crush!

Now, that's exercising some Girl Power!

Romance Is Not Random!

So how do you start to build that strong foundation for true love?

Just like with a friendship, you have to get to know each other's likes, dislikes, interests, fears and hobbies. You met each other because you had *something* in common—like a mutual friend, playing sports, same religion, same neighborhood, same job, same volunteer work—so that's a great place to start building a relationship. Start out by exploring that one thing you *know* you have in common. If it's a relationship that can turn into more than a crush, your question, "What position are you playing this season?" will soon turn into deeper conversations about the disappointment of losing and the elation of winning games, about teamwork and friendships among athletes, and about dreams of careers or colleges.

Once you figure out that you and your crush have things in common, it's important to get to know more and more about him. You'll also want to know about his family and family traditions. Most of all, you'll begin to understand his values. **And knowing your crush's values is important because "true loves" are not just randomly thrown together.** It takes two people with shared hopes and dreams and values to become true loves. So if a crush has become a boyfriend, and you're practicing how to move a boyfriend to the true love column, you have to know his values.

There are a million more things you can learn about your boyfriend. As you get to know these little things about him, you'll be learning whether this person is someone you can trust and be honest with about your own feelings. Enjoy getting to know your boyfriend—it's one of the most special parts of being a teenager! You could:

- Go with each other to school games, plays, concerts, volunteer activities.
- Swap favorite CDs.
- Learn each other's favorite things, like music groups, color, sports, books.
- Talk about great jobs to have when you are adults.
- Discuss what you will major in at college or what college you want to go to.

- Describe your dream vacations to each other.
- Go swimming, go hiking, play tennis, jump on the trampoline, shoot hoops, or pull out a pack of cards or a board game.
- Volunteer together in a community organization.
- Watch each other's favorite movie, even if it's not one you'd pick for yourself.
- Get to know each other's parents.
- Hang out with him around his brothers and sisters or best friends.
- Discuss or debate issues (i.e., the pros and cons of the new uniform policy at school or bigger issues like abortion or the death penalty) to challenge your thoughts and beliefs and see where each of you stands.

If you find you're still hanging out with him and feel comfortable trusting him, then you can start to share more intimate feelings and thoughts.

Think of some other things that you think would be fun to do with a boyfriend:

Think of some things you would want to know about him:

Getting **Closer** to Your Boyfriend (or True Love?)

You may have spent time getting to know your boyfriend, his family, his values, his likes, dislikes, goals and dreams, and now you might be feeling like he's a candidate for true love. You know lots of intimate things about him (that just means close, private, personal things), and now you might feel like being more *physically* intimate.

Getting to know a person intimately doesn't mean you have to have sex with him, but **you should be able to talk about it.** Physical closeness involves a lot more than sexual intercourse, so you need to be able to talk about *everything:* kissing, touching and sex. Boyfriends and girlfriends who have a plan and set boundaries for physical contact are more likely to stick to what's comfortable and not do something in the heat of the moment that they didn't plan on!

Can We Talk?

So how do you make a plan? You *have* to talk about it. Learning to communicate is a huge part of respecting each other. We know it's

uncomfortable, embarrassing and all that. But it has to be done to protect yourself and your boyfriend from letting physical things go too far.

If you are finding that talking about sexual things is really difficult,
start the conversation by talking about characters you saw on TV or in a
movie or maybe about what's going on between boyfriends and girlfriends at your school. That lets you get your ideas about what's okay in
teen relationships "out in the open." It will also help you and your
boyfriend start talking about what's okay in your relationship. But if you
can't talk, or he won't talk, *your* relationship is definitely not ready to
become physical!

"The talk" is tough, but once you have set your boundaries, it can be
totally fun! **Physical touch is a natural part of developing a relationship,** and part of your job as a teen is to practice these relationship things.

Don't Feel Pressured!

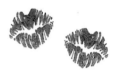

The teen world today is different from when your mom and dad were
hanging out in middle school and high school. Sex was rarely even mentioned in most households, and TV was as clean as church.

Sexual images and references are everywhere now—music videos, TV,
magazines, billboards, and blue jeans and T-shirt ads. The message today
is that sex is just something you do, regardless of your relationship or
responsibility or age. The result is that too many kids today feel pressure
to go straight to oral sex or sexual intercourse before a relationship even

really develops. **It leaves a lot of kids confused about being intimate.**

Just as there are a million ways to get to know your boyfriend, there are just as many ways to get to know each other physically without "going all the way." Adults call it *petting.* "Light" petting is holding hands, hugging and kissing lightly on the lips. You can also enjoy nonsexual stuff like a great back rub, a shoulder massage or a foot rub. (Foot rub? That would really take some strong feelings to rub the

feet of some guys we know! Peeeyooo!) "Heavy" petting is deeper kissing, French kissing and touching each other's genitals or breasts, either through clothing, under the clothes or undressed. Too often, heavy petting leads to sex if you don't set limits and stick by them.

You and your boyfriend *have* to be able to tell each other what feels good, what's appropriate and okay with you, and what you consider going too far. It can be awkward and a tough decision . . . but if you don't talk about it, you'll never be clear about your decisions and can easily get carried away "in the heat of the moment," especially if your guy is pushy.

And pushy guys are all about what feels good for *them.* They are all about getting what *they* want, and they'll keep pushing and pushing you until they get it. If it's not what YOU want, you need to **set clear limits.** Speak up fast and loud and tell him to STOP. Otherwise, you'll end up feeling bad about the experience and losing respect for yourself . . . we won't even talk about his respect for you, because there isn't any if he pushes you beyond what you are comfortable with. He is *definitely not* a true love. He's not even worthy of being a boyfriend.

So When Does a Boyfriend Become a True Love?

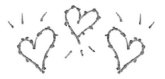

Now there's a tough one.

There are zillions of poems, songs, descriptions and explanations written about love. People talk about love all the time—and they associate it with things like your school, your country, music or art. There is also love for people like your family, your friends and unknown people in need all over the world. We even say we "love" something like an ice cream flavor, a girlfriend's shoes or a movie, when we mean that we really, really, really *like* it.

L   But what we're talking about here is **capital L, real, live, soul-mate romantic love.** This is the kind that leads people to get married and take care of each other for better and worse, for richer or poorer, for life. Rarely is true love something a teenager, even a mature one, actually experiences. But it IS something you work toward during the trial-and-error phase of crushes and first (and second and third . . .) boyfriends.

Here's our favorite description of it:

> *Love is patient and kind. Love isn't jealous and doesn't brag. It isn't rude or crude. Love is honest and trusting; it seeks the truth and looks out for the best interests of others. Love doesn't hold grudges, but gives second chances. Love is hopeful and long lasting and totally, incredibly awesome (taken from 1st Corinthians 13 with our own two cents thrown in).*

Learning about true love also means that you are preparing yourself for "Mr. Right" before you even meet him. You are determining your values so you will recognize a guy who shares values with you. You are developing your own plan for sexual involvement with crushes, boyfriends, your true love and the one you might marry.

You are also becoming more and more independent, more of your own individual with strong opinions, talents, interests, goals and dreams. True love means he respects your individuality and you respect his. You encourage each other to "be yourself." You encourage each other to do things with family and friends independent of each other.

True love means making and respecting sexual boundaries and being able to say no to sex when that is what is healthy for you. Besides, true love lasts forever, right? So remember, **you have lots of time.** Enjoy the long process of growing and learning more about each other as you develop and mature.

Healthy **Relationships**

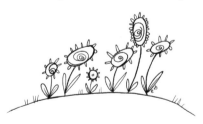

Think about true love and boyfriends. Every now and then a boyfriend might turn into a true love, but too many times, crushes or boyfriends turn out to be not so wonderful. Look at the following scenes and decide whether it is a sign of a healthy (on-the-way-to-true-love) or an unhealthy (never-gonna-get-there) relationship. Why do you think that?

Healthy	The Scenario . . .	Unhealthy
	He wants you with him all the time and gets angry if you want to spend time with your friends.	
	You feel comfortable talking to him about what you do and don't feel comfortable with sexually.	
	He makes all the decisions about where the two of you hang out and what you do.	
	You want to introduce him to all of your family.	
	You feel like he doesn't listen to the things you talk about, but he talks about himself all the time.	
	He gets in a fight after school with another guy who was flirting with you.	
	You feel angry when he tells you that he doesn't like holding hands in public.	
	He respects your need for privacy.	
	When you are hanging out in a group of friends, he gets a laugh out of "making fun of you" in front of everyone.	
	You tell your girlfriends every move he makes and the secrets he shares with you.	
	He does thoughtful things for you, and is respectful to your parents.	
	You feel like you need to impress him by buying and wearing certain clothes, even though they're not really "you."	
	You can talk to him about your fears or your beliefs or things that matter to you.	

Sometimes a guy is fun and cute and great about letting you be yourself, but he's lacking in other areas, like he may not be so cool around your parents or your friends. Guys are guys, **which means they aren't perfect.** So you don't have to hold yours up to an unreachable standard. But we do think that girls with Girl Power should be able to spot a good guy when they meet one (or as they get to know one), and can pick out a bad one, too.

Red Flags

And there *are* some bad ones out there. Ever heard of "red flags"? Red flags are big-time warnings, the equivalent of a red card in soccer, meaning "out of the game—*now!*" In relationships, you have to watch for red flags. Here's a list of red flags to help clue you in to an unhealthy relationship should you hook up with a bad, or even dangerous, guy. These are things that should be a deal breaker, no excuses allowed . . . out of the dating game—*now!*

 Is he overly jealous? (Remember, love is not jealous, so don't fool yourself into thinking he just likes you SOOO much if he gets jealous too easily.)

Does he get angry if you even talk to another guy?

Does he make you feel guilty if you do things with your friends or your family instead of him?

Does he use crude or disrespectful language when talking about girls or women in general?

Is he mean to animals?

Does he like to start fights or act like he will?

Does he blame you when he gets angry?

Is he EVER physically rough?

Does he use insulting words toward you or your friends?

Does he embarrass you in public?

Does he push you to do things sexually that you are not ready for?

Does he cheat or steal or use drugs?

Protecting Yourself

Some of this sounds scary. We don't want to scare you about relationships, but we do want you to know what can be lurking out there. Plus, if you want to figure out what true love is like, it helps to know what it's *not* like.

We're sure you know by now that some guys out there are "real losers," and we can't always control or stay away from them. **Nobody can protect herself from all bad things,** but you can keep yourself out of some risky and dangerous situations. As you gain more and more independence, this list of ways to protect yourself becomes more and more important:

- Get out of a relationship that has a red flag.
- Never accept a ride from a guy or man you don't know *very* well.
- Never experiment with drugs or alcohol around guys.
- Never agree to go alone to a guy's apartment, room or house.
- Don't accept a drink from someone if you don't know him well or aren't sure where it came from.
- Never, ever agree to go by yourself to meet someone in person whom you have met on the Internet.
- Do not give away any personal information on the Internet that would allow someone to locate you (name, address, phone number, school, location of after-school activities, etc.).

Enjoy Your Boyfriend

Now that we've gotten the "evil boyfriend" information out of the way, let's get back to the good guys. There are lots of them out there! If you are spending time getting to know guys' interests, talents and values, it will be easy to pick out the good ones. And the good ones are guys who can be friends and boyfriends!

When you find a good guy, **boyfriends can be a blast!** We still remember the first time our boyfriends surprised us and held our hands, the first time we slow danced and the first kisses we ever had. These are all occasions and feelings to cherish. We bet you'll remember them for a lifetime, too, so enjoy your boyfriend no matter what age you are, just make sure you stay in control!

Crushes

Crushes can be sort of strange and unexpected, too. Like when you have a crush on an older guy you might not even know, or maybe a teacher or a coach or the drummer from the local high school rock band. Or, of course, celebrities— with all their glitz and glamour and sex appeal—might infatuate you. Girls can even have a kind of "crush" on another girl, too. That doesn't mean you are gay. **A crush is just someone you idealize and want to be around,** someone you want to know more about, someone who sometimes makes you do silly things. As you get to know them better (if you do—sometimes you never even meet the person!), a crush may turn into a good friend (guy or girl) or a boyfriend.

The **End**

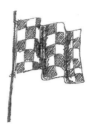

Of course the flip side of the fun of boyfriends is the fizzle. As a middle or high schooler, you'll learn that all good romances (and hopefully the bad ones!) will come to an end; it's part of this trial-and-error phase of growing up. You will develop new and different interests or realize that there are lots of other "fish in the sea." And you should! This is the natural course of things for teens. But sorry to say, that doesn't make it any easier when the breakup happens. The old-school song says it best, "Breaking up IS hard to do. . . ."

How do you handle it when your boyfriend "breaks your heart"? Do you hate him, become spiteful and talk bad about him to all your friends? We hope not. How do you break it to him when 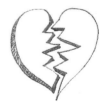 you're the one calling it quits? Get a friend to do your dirty work for you? Just start giving him the cold shoulder while you flirt with other guys? We hope not. If your relationship is based on respect and friendship in the first place (and we hope it is), then **a breakup should be done with respect,** too. It's still gonna hurt, but if you do it right—in a way that is gentle and gives as many honest reasons as you can—then your friendship will survive. Even though guys try not to show it, they have feelings and they get broken hearts, too.

Remember, this is still trial-and-error time. You're going to make some mistakes (and he is too!), so think about what worked and what didn't, what hurt more than it should have and what you might be able to do differently next time, so that breaking up gets easier. Maybe these tips from experienced heartbreakers will help:

- If you're the one doing the breaking up, and you see it coming, give a few **gentle hints** to lead up to it.
- **Be honest!!** Don't make up excuses or blame him for things that aren't true just to make it easier for you. It'll backfire in the end.
- **Go easy** on him. No need to spread rumors, burn bridges or rub noses in the dirt.
- If he's the one who calls it off, **don't let your hurt turn into anger.** Spite never healed a broken heart.
- **Be patient with yourself.** You WILL get over it, all in good time. Use it as an opportunity to reconnect with family, girlfriends or guy friends you may have ignored more than usual when you were busy with your boyfriend.
- If he starts going out with one of your good friends, **try to be understanding.** Keep your friendship and their relationship separate. It's not about you anymore!

The bottom line is, how you handle a breakup situation says a lot about how you handle relationships in general. Your level of maturity, honesty, trustworthiness and kind-heartedness is an important part of your reputation among guys and girls. Nobody said it'd be easy, but **it's always easier to do it right!!**

Choices to Make!

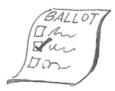

You are not likely to find true love in your teen years, especially your early teen years. But you do get to **have some fun practicing at true love.** You do get to feel the excitement of crushes, enjoy getting to know guys as friends and love interests, and feel the first urges of sexual desire.

This is a time full of choices *you* get to make. And **making choices that protect your body, your heart and your emotions will increase your power**—your Girl Power!

You get to choose how you will get to know a crush better. You get to choose what physical things you will do with a boyfriend. You get to choose the good guys and leave the bad guys behind at the first sign of a "red flag." Remember that you are "in training" for the day when you will meet your real true love. Learn, remember and enjoy every minute of it!

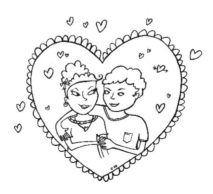

12

When Is What Okay?

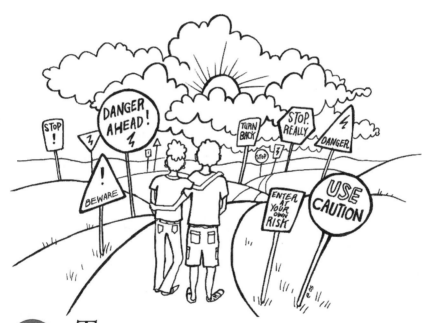

This is an awesome, powerful, exciting time of your life. As a young teen, your body is changing, your feelings are changing, your thoughts are changing, your relationships are changing, guys are changing. You *are* up for the challenge, aren't you?

Remember those two big tasks you must complete before you become an adult? The first is becoming independent. The second is figuring out "who you are." In this chapter we will work on figuring out who you are. That means figuring out what you *value.*

Values are things you consider important. They are principles, ideas and beliefs that help you make decisions. **Each person should live her life according to her values.** And if you are true to your values, your values will guide your behavior.

It works like this. If you value a clean environment, you don't pollute. If you value honesty, you tell the truth. If you value your health, you don't smoke cigarettes. It's easy to stick to your values when it's convenient, like when telling the truth doesn't get you in any trouble, or the trash can is right next to you, or your friends gag every time they smell cigarette smoke.

But **values are things that don't change even if they aren't easy to follow.** So to be true to your values, you'll have to keep the environment clean even when the trash can is all the way on the other side of the park. You'll have to tell the truth even when it makes you look bad. You'll have to turn down cigarettes even when the most gorgeous guy in school flips out a pack and offers you a smoke.

Sticking to your values when it's hard is called *building character.* **And it's not easy!** How much fun is it to tell the truth when you are the one who will get in trouble? Or lug your trash all the way across the park when everybody else is darting off to the basketball court? Or turn down cigarettes when the cool girls say it looks sophisticated?

It's difficult. But at the end of the day, you can look yourself in the mirror and say, "You know, that was tough, but I stuck to my values and *that* feels good!" It's a choice you make, tough or easy. And it's a great way to practice your Girl Power!

What Do I Value?

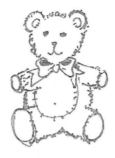

All of this is to say that values are important! They are the foundation of that deep question, "Who am I?" And you are at the perfect age to start answering that question! You don't have to know for certain what you want to be when you grow up, where you will go to college or who you will marry. But you *do* have to start thinking about how you want to act and what you think is important. You *do* have to think about what you value.

Deep stuff, huh? But you really already know a lot about values. Your parents, your grandparents, your other family members and other caregivers have taught you values your entire life. You have also learned from teachers, religious leaders and coaches along the way. Take some time and think about the values you have already learned. Pay attention. Write them down. **Keep a list.**

Remember, values are ideas and principles plus action. So if your parents value education, they make sure you complete your assignments every day and discuss your subjects with you. If your grandmother values the arts, she takes you to art exhibits, concerts and recitals. If your religious leader values loving your neighbor, she takes you to the soup kitchen to serve people less fortunate than you. Bet you've learned more than you thought!

The **Friend** Factor

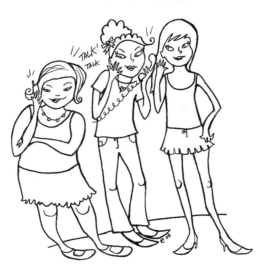

You are still learning a lot about values from the adults in your life, but as we said at the beginning of this book, things are changing! Now that you are an adolescent, you are paying more attention to your friends and other teens who may not have the same values you do. **Your friends with other values will challenge what you believe in.** That's when it's most important to understand your own values. If you are not sure what your values are, look to your family and the people who care about you to help you decide. Check out that list you've been keeping!

There are some values that should be universal. That means that most everyone in the universe agrees with them. Obviously, there will always be crazy, mixed-up people, like criminals and tyrant leaders who don't fit in to "our" universe, and that's why they seem crazy and mixed up, because they don't follow the values that normal people live by. For example, we can probably say that most people value the Earth, fairness, justice, safety, freedom and relationships with others.

There are other values that depend on the individual and are neither right nor wrong. What's important is what your values lead you to do. For example, a lot of people value money. This can sometimes cause problems, like if they start to steal to get more money. But valuing money can be good, too. Think about the wealthy person who donates large amounts of money to build houses for homeless people. That's cool, and nobody would say she was a bad person for valuing money.

Is it bad to value things? Valuing things is called being **materialistic**. It's usually used in a negative way, but it's not so bad if you don't let it control everything you do, and you have other values that keep it in check.

Let's say you really value your clothes and makeup. Are you a bad person? Nope. But what if you value clothes and makeup so much that you won't be friends with someone who doesn't wear the "right" clothes? Now that's being shallow. You'd miss out on a lot of great friends if that's all you based your friendships on. If you value clothes, makeup AND honesty, independence and kindness, then you're working with a **fuller set of values** that will make you a happier person and a better friend to others.

These examples show that there are lots of different types of things that we value. We can put them into categories to make it easier to understand. You can value:

People and relationships—friends, family members, crushes and boyfriends, pets (sure, pets can be considered people, but if you think about it, it's probably the way your pet makes you feel and depends on you and even loves you that you value most)

Actions—horseback riding, drawing, sports, playing or listening to music

Ideas—honesty, trust, loyalty, humor, fairness, popularity, independence
Things—books, stuffed animals, bicycle, special piece of jewelry, your hair

Think about your values and the values of the people you know.

	Me	My Best Buds	My Parents
People			
Things			
Actions			
Ideas			

Do you see similarities in this chart? We bet you do! That's because **most people choose friends based on similar values and beliefs.** You might have some differences from your parents, but they have definitely influenced you.

But **Why?**

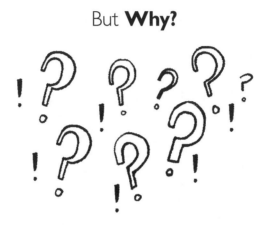

Now, remember we told you that you are old enough to start knowing WHY when your parents tell you what they think or want. **Let's think about your own whys.** Why do you value the things you listed?

So where are we going with this? As you enter the world of crushes and romance, **you need to have a very strong idea about what you value in relationships.** Your friends and family have helped you make that list of values. Now it's time to think ahead about what you would value in your relationship with your true love. Are there certain things and ideas you dream of having in your relationship with your true love?

Some of them will be simple. Let's look at the categories:

People and relationships: Duh, that's your true love you have to value.

Actions: Spending time together in nature, studying together, going to a concert together, riding bikes together, gazing into each other's eyes.

Ideas: Honesty, loyalty, trust, respect.

Things: You might value the bracelet he gave you or a note he wrote you.

What else? What other things are really important in a relationship? Think hard . . . how about your body and his body?! That includes your physical and emotional health.

Value Your **Body!** It's the Only One You've Got!

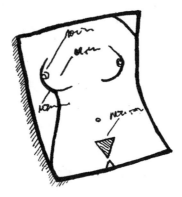

But wait . . . do YOU value your body? That's a tough one. We know that a lot of girls DON'T feel good about their bodies. WHY? Is it because magazines have made them feel they don't look like toothpicky models?

What about you? **Do you feel okay about your body?** Have kids at school told you your body isn't good enough? Are you taking care of your body like you should by eating healthy (veggies, water, avoiding fast food and junk food), exercising (sports, walking, getting off the couch and away from the computer), and protecting it from harm (wearing helmets, seat belts, avoiding drugs and alcohol, abstaining from sex or protecting yourself against pregnancy and sexually transmitted infections)?

If you don't take care of your body, who will? If you don't take care of it, you lose respect for it. **What a shame!** Our bodies are amazing things. Think about the five senses (touching, smelling, seeing, tasting, hearing) and the things like music, nature, textures, food and beauty they allow you to experience. Remember all the stuff about growing a baby? Your body is miraculous and helps you DO incredible stuff! **Bodies are powerful!**

Respect your body, and make sure your boyfriend shares that value. Your boyfriend will never become your true love unless he shares your values. If you have a boyfriend who doesn't share your values and pushes you to do things that you are not comfortable with, it's time for **the big dump, the breakup, the drop off.** You can never truly be close to someone who doesn't share your most important values.

It's never easy, but it's a rule we all need to live by: Choose boyfriends who respect your body! Now *that's* a decision that gives us girls power and strength!

Decision Time

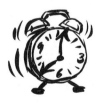

Okay. So what happens when you've stuck by your rule to choose a boyfriend who shares your values and respects your body? Good job! He's looking like Mr. Perfect, true-love-wannabe. You feel emotionally intimate because you've gotten to know each other. You are definitely having those warm, tingly feelings of sexual desire. It's thrilling, exciting . . . and overwhelming. Yikes! **Where do you go now?**

A big part of growing up is figuring out how you will handle situations that involve being close with another person. That means figuring out what you expect of yourself when it comes to having sex and doing things that are sexual. Maybe you haven't really thought about it yet, but you need to start deciding when it will be okay to do some sexual things.

Why now? Now, because you are **smart enough** to figure out what is important to you. Now, because you are becoming **independent enough** to make good decisions. Now, because you are growing up and **becoming the type of girl who sticks to her values in lots of different situations**—when it's easy *and* when it's hard.

Plan It Now

It's time for you to start thinking about your future and making some promises to yourself . . . maybe you can even make some promises to your future true love. Isn't that dreamy? If you decide and promise yourself now, you'll be more likely to **stick with those promises,** even in the "heat of a romantic moment."

Girls who have a plan about when it is okay to have sex are more likely to stick with that decision and not let some smooth-talking guy change their plans. There is a lot of power in having a plan!

So, What's Your Plan Gonna Be?

You'll hear lots of different answers, especially to the question of when it is okay to "go all the way" or have sexual intercourse. You'll hear things like:

- When you are married
- When you are dating steady
- When you are 18 years old
- When you have been dating a boy for one year (or maybe six months or even three months)
- Whenever you feel like it
- When a guy says he loves you

Talk about those mixed messages!

Your plan for physical closeness with a guy will involve a lot more than just sexual intercourse, but let's start there since it is the most important decision.

Why Wait?

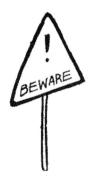

There are plenty of good reasons to wait to have sex: We're going to sound like parents for a minute (and uh . . . we are parents), but here goes. If you wait until you are an adult in a mature, long-term, committed relationship before you have sex, then:

- There is **less emotional "baggage,"** such as guilt, disappointment and fear.
- You will have a **more mature relationship** before you have sex.
- You will have **better sex** with your eventual husband when you don't have memories of sex with other guys.
- You can **accept pregnancy** as a consequence and become a parent when you will be excited and prepared for it.

Now we're going to sound like **doctors** for a minute (remember, we are doctors, too). More good reasons to delay sexual activity are:

- Girls who have sex at a younger age tend to have **more sexual partners** during their lifetimes.
- You will have **less risk** for cervical cancer if you have fewer sexual partners. Every new guy you have sex with increases your chance of getting a virus that can cause cervical cancer.

- The younger you are when you have sex, the higher your risk for **sexually transmitted infections.** Infections can cause infertility, cancer, pain, even death.
- You can't get pregnant if you don't have sex. **Pregnancy** in middle school or high school is not what most girls want or need.

And finally we're just going to sound like **girlfriends** (we *are* female and we *do* care). More good reasons to delay sexual activity are:

- Young guys **aren't typically interested** in the relationship as much as they are interested in getting sexual experience or pleasure.
- Many young guys **don't feel the same emotional** attachment with sex that girls typically feel. The emotional part seems to come at a later age for guys.
- Teen boys can be great friends, but they are often awkward or self-centered when it comes to sex and making girls enjoy the sexual experience. They make themselves feel good, but they **don't really understand** how to help you feel good and enjoy sex.

It's a Big Deal!

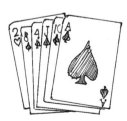

Sex *is* a big deal. It can be awesome with the right person, but it takes a mature relationship that most girls don't experience until they are adults, so why waste it?

So what do you do in the meantime? **The wait can be fun!** Once you have a romantic interest, someone you trust and want to be with, you'll need to decide how far you will go. If the intimate feelings are there, there are lots of different things you can do to physically enjoy each other or to show affection.

There are some **risk-free things** that are fun, like holding hands, hugging, giving a back rub or shoulder massage, and playing with each other's hair. Things like this allow you to spend time comfortably together without feeling pressured to do sexual things.

There are some activities that are more intimate but still **not so risky,** like kissing. Some teens can kiss for hours without going any further. Before you even think about going further, spend some time perfecting your kissing skills. That can be fun.

The thing is, once you go past the kissing stage, **it can be really, really, really hard to stop!** Your body is made so that all the touching gets you more and more sexually excited. In fact, when men and women *plan* to have sex, that's exactly what they do to get their bodies ready for sexual intercourse. Remember the foreplay stuff?

So if you don't want to go all the way . . . some types of touching, massaging and kissing each other's bodies is really confusing. Your brain knows that you have decided not to have sexual intercourse, but you are doing things that make your brain want to tell your body to go for it! See how important it is to **decide when you will stop** before things get all hot and heavy?!

How Do You Decide?

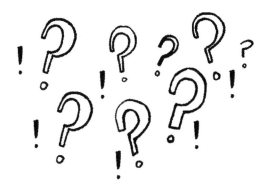

Setting your sexual boundaries is important, *really* important. It puts you in control of your body, your emotions and your relationships. It's one of those choices that can be tough, but if you **stick to your boundaries,** you can be proud at the end of the day (or night).

The time to decide on your boundaries is:

- When you have time to **think**
- When you have a chance to **discuss it** with trusted adults and friends, if you want to
- **Before** you get in a sexual situation
- Maybe even **before** you have a boyfriend

The time to decide on your boundaries is *not:*

- Before you have time to think
- When you feel pressured by a boyfriend or your girlfriends
- When you are already in a sexual situation (like heavy kissing or touching)

Now, down to the specifics! Look at the following list and spend some time thinking about when you think the activity will be okay *for you.*

When Is It Okay To . . .

- Hold hands?
- Go out together in a group?
- Hug?
- Kiss on the lips?
- Go out on a date alone?
- French kiss?
- Let your boyfriend touch your breasts through your clothes?
- Let your boyfriend touch your bare breasts?
- Touch your boyfriend's penis?
- Undress in front of each other?
- Have oral sex?
- Have sexual intercourse?
- Have a baby together?

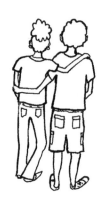

Some of these are easy answers. You can hold hands with your boyfriend any time, risk free! Other answers are tough and will be unique to your values and comfort level.

With most of your boyfriends and even with some guys you think are true loves, you'll **never** get to a lot of the things on this list, **and that, my friend, is good!** Many of these things should be reserved for adult, real, live true loves and some for the person you marry.

What's Okay **When**?

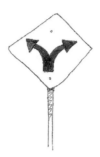

You have to ask yourself:

- What is **healthiest for my body?** (Check out the "we're sounding like doctors" list on page 226 and 227.)
- What is **healthiest for my emotions?** (Check out the "we're sounding like parents and girlfriends" lists on pages 226 and 227.)
- What things will I do with a **crush?** A boyfriend?
- **How do I know** he's a crush? A boyfriend?
- What will I do with a **true love?**
- **How do I know** he's a true love?
- Will I **save something** special for marriage?

Boyfriends and crushes are pretty easy to figure out. They give you that twitterpated (did you ever see *Bambi*?), butterflies-in-the-stomach feeling, even though you may not know them well (or even know them at all!). **True loves can be trickier.** You have the same butterfly feelings about a true love, but you also have to know a true love well. You have to share values, time and experiences together.

Believe it or not, you may think you have many "true loves" in the next ten years. You might think one's a true love, but then you get to know him better and find out things you don't like. Or maybe you just develop a crush on another guy, and suddenly your former "true love" doesn't give you the butterflies anymore.

That's all okay. Just remember that when you decide what sexual things you will do with a true love, if it's too much, too soon, you'll just end up embarrassed and feeling disappointed. **We don't know any girl or woman who has ever regretted waiting to have sex.** But we see tons who are disappointed and mad at themselves for having sex too soon with someone they thought was a true love but didn't turn out to be the one. Chances are you will not end up marrying the boyfriend you have at age fourteen, so wait it out. Get to know what you like and don't like in a relationship, but save the sex for much later.

It's Too Late for **Me**

What if you're reading this thinking, "Oh, great. This doesn't even apply to me. I've already let a guy touch my breasts/touched a guy's penis/had sexual intercourse. I didn't have a good plan before, and now I've blown it."

Hey! It's okay! And we promise you it's *not* too late.

We all make mistakes. You are not alone. Most young teens are not satisfied with their first sexual experience. You didn't have a plan then, but you can make one now! Just because you've gone farther than you wanted to doesn't mean that you have to go that far with every guy you date from now on.

Reset your boundaries. Make a promise to yourself to stick to your plan. Learn from your mistakes and make changes to protect your body and your emotions. This is where that strong character you have developed by choosing values and sticking with them comes in. Once you have crossed a boundary it will be hard to reset. We know that. But we also know that sticking to your promises to yourself is important even when it's hard. **And we know you can do it!**

Now **This** Should Be Interesting . . .

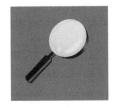

If you really want to have some fun, give the "When Is It Okay?" list to your parents and have them fill it out. There's an interesting conversation!

Talk with your mom or another trusted adult female about this stuff. See if you can get your dad to talk with you about it. **Dads have important opinions, too!** Are your answers different from your parents'? Ask your parents not only WHEN but WHY. Make them explain their reasons for their answers. Do they make sense? Believe it or not, parents know more than you think about this stuff.

Parents probably feel **awkward** talking with you about it, but they'll have some great advice if you'll hear them out. You don't need to know if or when your parents did all this stuff (ewwwww!), but their answers will be based on what they have learned from their own experiences and life in general.

But, What If . . . ?

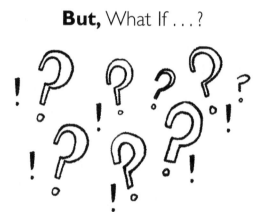

Everyone makes mistakes sometimes, so we have to talk about the what ifs.

Hopefully, we've made the point that for humans, sex is not supposed to be *just* for reproducing. It's also not supposed to be something you try *just* because you're curious. You know by now that **sex is *powerful*** in many ways. **It can be a wonderful, intimate experience that two people share. It can also be a very disappointing, embarrassing, and even scary experience if it happens too soon or in the wrong relationship.**

The disappointing and scary part can come in many ways. We're doctors; we hear these stories almost every day! Consider the following **real-life examples:**

- A 14-year-old girl has sex with her guy "friend" because she is **just curious** to see what it is like. She ends up pregnant.
- A 26-year-old woman can't enjoy sex with her husband because she

had sex as a young teenager in a bad relationship and has **bad memories** that get in the way of her enjoyment.

- A 15-year-old girl goes on a date with her crush, a very popular soccer player at her school who is 17. He starts kissing her, then talks her into giving him oral sex even though **she didn't really want to.** He never calls again but tells all his friends at school what they did.
- A 16-year-old sneaks out of her house to go to a party her parents didn't want her to go to. She drinks a lot of beer and has sex for the **first time** ever with a guy she doesn't really know very well.
- A 14-year-old girl and her boyfriend start kissing and get really sexually excited. They touch each other through their clothes. Then they pull their clothes off and touch each other's naked bodies. They've said they wouldn't have sex, but in the **heat of the moment** they both really want to. And they do.

You can see from these true stories why a plan is so important and powerful for girls! Every single girl in these stories either did something she *really didn't want to* do or suffered a negative consequence from having sex too early and in the wrong relationship.

And you can also see why you need to work really hard to help yourself stick to your plan. If you want to **stick by your promise to yourself to respect your body,** you also have to keep yourself out of situations that make it really hard to do that (like drinking alcohol and taking drugs, being alone with a guy you're not sure you can trust, going "so far" that it's hard to stop). Those are things you are in control of. Those are decisions you get to make. You have the power and the choice to learn from bad decisions and to **make better ones in the future.** That's another way to show your Girl Power!

Some **Good** News about **Guys**

We know it kind of sounds like guys want nothing but power over you or to get in your pants, like they have no self-control, like they are only worried about themselves and their sexual desires and not you. Well, there *is* good news! There are **guys out there who put you before themselves.** They are the kind of guys who may even want to stop sooner than you do. They are the ones who will stop and make a good

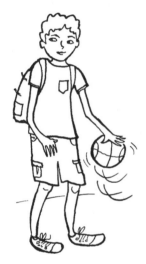

decision for you even when you are thinking about going further. They are the ones who will remind you that you both decided to stop at the French kiss, and they will respect that decision and make you stick with it!

Those are the guys to look for. You'll know them by the way they respect girls and women. They don't act all nice-mannered to fool the teachers, then harass girls in the hallway. They might be quiet, they might be loud, they might play in a band, they might be good at goofing around, they might be jocks or nerds or drama kings . . . but **the good ones know respect**—for you and for themselves and others. See one? **Get to know him.** It takes time to decide whether he is worthy of YOU.

Power in Planning

If there is one single thing we want you to remember from this chapter, it's that there is **power in the plan!**

Values and boundaries are super important, so do your best to "stay in bounds!" especially when you have your first (or next!) boyfriend. The closer you get to feeling true love, the harder it will be to stick to your plan. Because now you are talking about a real live guy—a guy you are attracted to and really want to be physically close to. It's not that theoretical "someday" boyfriend you probably had in mind when you set your boundaries. Enjoy your new sexuality, **enjoy being emotionally intimate, kiss, look sexy if you want to, but it doesn't mean you have to have sex.** Once you are ready for sex, you will also understand the importance of having a plan to discuss it with your true love and make sure you protect yourself against pregnancy and infections.

We'll say it again: Girls who have a plan are less likely to do sexual things they really don't want to do. Sticking to your plan is easier if your boyfriend respects you. And true loves *always* respect you. It will be awkward talking to your boyfriend about sexual things and boundaries. But getting the relationship right requires communication, **lots of communication.** And you can do it!

Just remember, values stay the same no matter what situation you are in. If it was good for you before you met your boyfriend, it's still good for you today. **Promises to yourself are worth keeping even if it's hard to do.** Be strong! You are definitely worth it!

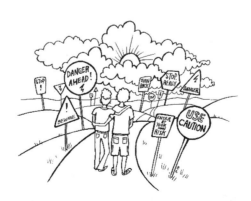

PART FOUR

Growing Real Girl Power

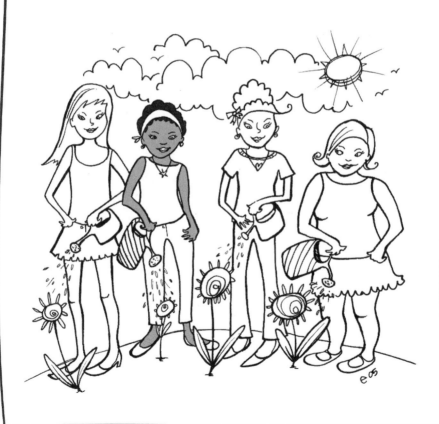

13

Get Your Girl Power On!

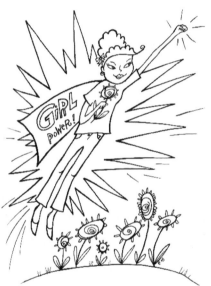

By now, we hope that you have seen a glimpse and felt a **pulse of power**—the power that is within you. It's an amazing power that will bring you so many good things and protect you from bad things if you learn how to use it. Why do so many teen girls feel *powerless* over so much of what goes on in their lives? We think it's because they haven't discovered the power that they carry within them—**real live Girl Power.**

So you, whether you have recognized it or not, have amazing power. Not just power related to sex and sexuality, but a bigger power that comes with the ability to make **choices that matter.** You have the ability to choose how you want to be seen, who you trust, when you are ready for intimacy, and importantly, you have the power to say no to things that aren't in your best interest.

Now, when we combine the words **power** and **sex,** a lot of people get the wrong impression. People talk about using sex for power or using sex to get what you want. That's not *good* power. It's just *using* something powerful to **manipulate** others. Your sexuality is something special that should be treasured and respected, not abused. Sexuality just happens to be a very powerful thing that you have, whether you want it or not.

She Figured It Out

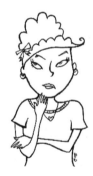

Remember that girl we talked about in chapter 2? The one with the Girl Power? The one who says she's sorry when she hurts a friend's feelings. The one who cuts her parents some slack even when she thinks they totally don't get it. The one who understands how her body works and can talk about it without getting too embarrassed. The one who makes a plan for her own sexual involvement and chooses a boyfriend who will respect her decisions. Yep, that one. The one everyone seems to look up to and respect.

She obviously figured out a lot of stuff for herself, a lot of the things we've been talking about. Things like:

- Using **words wisely**
- **Not giving any power away** to people who want to embarrass or use her

- **Listening to people who want what's good for her**—not TV, movies, music, magazines and advertisers that want what's best for them
- Choosing **friends who build her up** and don't tear her down—and being a good friend to others as well
- Recognizing that she is sexual and **can be sexy without "doing it"**
- **Talking, thinking and learning** about sexual things before she gets "in the heat of the moment" and does something she regrets
- Being **brave** enough to talk to boyfriends about her sexual boundaries—even when it's really awkward.
- Telling the **difference between** good boyfriends and bad boyfriends
- **Saving** some sexual things for her true love

Will it always be easy to make decisions and do things that help grow your Girl Power? Absolutely not. Sometimes it will feel great—the easiest decision you've ever made! Sometimes it will totally stink! Some people might even tell you you're stupid, afraid, freaky, **weird** and totally don't get it. **But when it stinks,** you have to remember that you are making decisions that are good for you for life . . . not just for the moment. It's hard work, but it pays off in the end.

It's like the girl who gets made fun of for shooting baskets every Saturday morning instead of going to the mall. The shooting isn't all that much fun, but then on Friday night, she fakes out the defense with two seconds to go and sinks a three-pointer to win the game. They called her boring when she was practicing, but she's a **hero** when her practice makes her win the game!

Growing your Girl Power takes practice too. And it lets you be a hero for life—a hero to yourself! **Too many girls grow impatient** in this work to grow Girl Power. They compromise their values because of it. Not good.

You Are Worth the Best

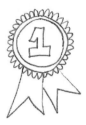

There is a lot of power that comes for waiting for the best, not just grabbing all the cheap stuff you can get as soon as it comes your way. And get ready, because sex will come your way during your teen years. **You have to be ready to handle it.** You have to be able to make and stick to a plan for sexual limits and behaviors that are healthy for you.

Patience and self-control pay off in the end; we promise! If you are making good choices and good decisions now (even though they may be difficult, other teens roll their eyes at you or boys may pressure you), you will look back not too far from now and see the power in the choices you made . . . the power in having a plan.

We're not just making it up. Every day we talk to young girls and women who are healthy and happy because they have stuck to a plan about sex and sexual stuff that feels right for them. They feel powerful and in control. And we also hear too many stories from girls who have made some serious mistakes because they didn't have a plan at all.

Things "just happened"—then there was a lot of regret and tears, sometimes even pregnancy or infections. Every time girls give away or allow someone else to "take" some of this power, it's a loss. Their power weakens, and they have to work hard to start to rebuild it. Fortunately, it **can** be built up again! They have to go back and **make some new choices that give them power and control.** And they have to stick to those choices and hold on to that power to let it grow.

Claim Your Girl Power

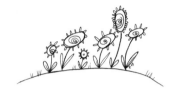

This whole power thing goes back way farther than women today. Since the beginning of time, civilizations have recognized that people have special opportunities in life to gain power. Periods of transition are times of especially great power! Think about some of the major transitions in a girl's life:

Birth—power to be on this Earth

Puberty—power to reproduce and create new life

Marriage—power to start a relationship that can create a family

Motherhood—power to shape a new life into something powerful

Menopause—power to share wisdom and see life from a very experienced perspective

Let's look at one of these life transitions to understand this power thing. It's a little touchy-feely and deep kind of stuff. **But it's true.**

Birth . . . yep, pretty powerful. Think of all the amazing potential newborn babies have. Even though they are totally dependent on other caregivers to feed them, get them around and nurture them . . . their **potential is limitless.** Somewhere, a baby is being born who will be a future president or an inventor or an Olympic champion or the biggest rock star the world has ever seen! On the other hand, babies are being born who will be haters, cheaters and criminals. So just because there is a lot of power in the birth transition . . . it doesn't always end up being *good power.* But birth is an opportunity for a new little human being to start **collecting power to become anything in the world.**

Now, let's get back to you and the power transition you're in right now.

You've Got Power!

So here you are at one of life's major transitions. You are making the transition from a child—through puberty and adolescence—into a young adult. **Can you feel the power? You should!**

A main purpose of puberty is to develop sexually. Sexual power is a mighty thing that a girl possesses. You aren't supposed to use it for bad things like controlling other people or making them jealous. You are supposed to **protect** that power and, then as you mature, **share** it with the one who has helped you protect it and who also respects and values it.

As a teen, you are developing your ability to appreciate your body, to enjoy sexual feelings and to develop meaningful relationships outside of your family. You have the potential to develop great respect for your sexuality and ability to reproduce. Now that's good power! You also have the potential to mess it up by having unintended pregnancies, by getting infections that can harm your ability to have babies if you want to in the future and by losing respect for how awesome sex can be in the right relationship. That would be bad power, right?

In our culture and in the human experience, sex is powerful. Don't let anyone talk you into believing that it's no big deal.

Power Thieves

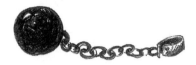

The more that you hold on to that special power within you, the stronger it can become. **Many people will try to take it away from you.** Some teenage boys and some adult men are always trying to take that power away from girls and women. They may do that by trying to become sexually involved too soon or by making comments that make you feel uncomfortable about your body or your sexuality. Same for some advertisers, magazines, movies and other girls—they will try to diminish your sexual power, to make it seem unimportant or not worth taking care of.

All we have to say is that THEY ARE WRONG! You have great power as a girl. They want a piece of it because you have an amazing and wonderful Girl Power! **If it weren't a big deal, nobody would want it or care about it.**

Protect Your Girl Power

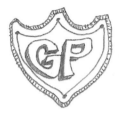

If you haven't yet, you will eventually begin to recognize the power. Once you notice how strong it is, you might want to use it to your benefit. Sometimes you *want* to give it away because:

- 🌀 You know it is **strong**.

- 🌀 It gets **attention**.

- 🌀 It seems **exciting**.

But be careful! **If you give it away too soon, it starts to decrease.** It becomes less and less and less. But if you hold on to it and **protect it and respect it, it will grow and grow and grow.** When you do find true love, your true love will also respect that power and help you to protect it. When the time is right to share it, it doesn't decrease when you release it . . . it grows! That's when intimacy and sex are great! It feels great physically, it feels great in your heart, and it feels powerful. With the right person, your sexual power and all this other power you've been growing is a **gift** for both of you.

It's important to keep that power within you until you know you have found true love. Depending on your values, that may mean marriage. Too many girls give it away in middle school or high school **when they**

don't really know that they have true love. Sex doesn't make true love. True love lasts, right? What's the rush? Don't give it away!

And if you've already given some of it away to guys who don't respect and protect you, you can stop! Just because you've made one (or two or three or twenty-five) mistakes, it doesn't mean you have to keep giving your power away over and over again. If you've felt that loss of power before, you know what we mean. Girls who have felt that power loss learn that **sex in the wrong relationship isn't worth the stress, the worry, the emotions and the physical risks.** But if you make new choices to protect yourself and your sexual power, you'll have something special to share when you do have true love. You can build your Girl Power back up!

People who try to take your power away from you aren't interested in you. They are just interested in stealing something special. The person who values your Girl Power, protects it and helps it grow wants what is best for you. He is interested in you. He knows that your Girl Power is special. **And he likes that!**

Take control of your body. Learn how it works. Make a plan for your sexual involvement. Protect and grow your Girl Power. Save it for yourself and true love. **Be Powerful!**

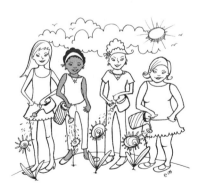

Acknowledgments

Girlology would have never blossomed like it has without some magical connections. We are so grateful for the special people who have been placed in our paths, particularly our energetic and hip editor Amy Hughes who has been wonderfully enthusiastic about *Girlology* since that first day at Starbucks. We would have never met her without another writer, Marcia Higgins White, who put us in the public eye. The other amazing connection occurred with Jennifer Craig, our legal eagle, Nikki and Abby at *Skirt!* magazine, and Sally Pascutti and Stephanie Hunt our intuitive wordsmiths. We know how these magical connections really occur, and we are grateful.

We are also indebted to many steadfast cheerleaders. Robin Berlinsky, Gina English, Carolyn Evans, Beth Rucker and Beth Cairns have provided great ideas and energy. We relied heavily on the awesome mom-daughter groups who provided critical review, insight and suggestions. They include Lyn, Rachel and Sarah Neil; Laura, Megan and Jamie Spinella; Susan Simonian and Katie Houle. We also appreciate the patience and support of our colleagues at Charleston Pediatrics and East Cooper Women's Center.

We'd each like to thank our parents for their unwavering support and tolerance of our "openness." We love you dearly. Our husbands, also tolerant and unconditionally loving, have been incredibly patient and encouraging. Thanks Michael and Steve for keeping it all together while cheering us on. Our daughters, Emily, Caroline, Ella, Anne Claire and Maehler, have been our inspiration. We hope each of you will grow up to be confident and secure with your power and not be embarrassed that your moms go around talking about puberty and sexuality.

Finally, we are most appreciative of the thousands of mothers who have trusted us to start important conversations with their daughters, and to the daughters who have taught us so much. Keep on talking!

About the Authors

In a casual conversation one day, Dr. Melisa Holmes, an ob-gyn and Dr. Trish Hutchison, a pediatrician, laughed about how often mothers seem to stiffen with fear when the topics of puberty and sexuality come up. "How do I start the conversation?" "What do I say?" "Can I just bring my child to you and let you give her *the talk*?" These questions are a daily occurrence in both of their offices. Fortunately, moms have come to the right place because Drs. Holmes and Hutchison are both passionate about helping girls feel good about and understand their changing bodies.

In over twenty years of combined experience as popular, overbooked physicians, Dr. Holmes and Hutchison have answered these questions innumerable times. Now they can't believe how much fun they have providing programs to families to help get these conversations started!

Since 2002, these physicians have developed two programs for mother-daughter pairs, a series of classes for older teens (males and females), and several programs for parents only. All of their classes fill up rapidly and each class generates a new group of waiting participants for the next program. The demand has spread far beyond their hometown of Charleston, South Carolina and beyond what these two practicing physicians can offer.

Dr. Holmes is a native of Atlanta, Georgia, a magna cum laude graduate of the University of Georgia, and a graduate of the Medical College of Georgia. Following her ob-gyn internship and residency at the Medical College of Virginia, Melisa joined the faculty at the Medical University of South Carolina (MUSC) in Charleston where she holds joint appointments in Obstetrics/Gynecology and Pediatrics, and has been named among the Best Doctors in America. During her twelve years of clinical practice, she was director of the MUSC Teen Clinic and founder and director of the Sexual Assault Follow-up Evaluation (SAFE) clinic. As a nationally recognized advocate for adolescent health, she has served on the American College of Obstetrics and Gynecology Committee on Adolescent Health Care, and the National Campaign to Prevent Teen Pregnancy. She has written numerous peer-reviewed scientific papers in the medical literature, as well as textbook chapters on a variety of subjects related to adolescent gynecology and care of the sexual assault victim. In the medical community, she is a nationally recognized speaker on topics of adolescent gynecology, teen sexuality, interpersonal violence, and other issues in women's health. Her daughter Emily has been a special consultant to *Girlology,* her middle daughter, Caroline, knows her time is coming soon, and her youngest, Ella (still a baby) will keep Dr. Holmes in touch with girls for a long time to come.

Dr. Hutchison is a South Carolina girl. She grew up in Rock Hill, graduated cum laude from the College of Charleston and earned her M.D. at the Medical University of South Carolina. After completing her Pediatrics internship and residency at Vanderbilt University in Nashville, Trish came back to Charleston, where she was in private practice for ten years. She currently practices in the Adolescent Medicine Department at MUSC where she directs Girls2Women, a young women's health center.

She, too, has been named among the Best Doctors in America. She developed her interest in adolescents during years of peer counseling and youth mentoring. Today, she continues to enjoy the challenges and rewards of adolescent medicine. In her community, her practice has always been full of adolescent girls and boys. She has an amazing way with teens and at the same time earns their parents unwavering respect and trust. She is recognized as a wonderful resource in her community for health-related issues, particularly related to growth and development, and sexuality and behavioral issues. Trish is actively involved in community service organizations and in her church. She has also participated in mission work delivering health care to children and adolescents, but she mostly likes sticking close to home, where her two girls, Anne Claire and Maehler, keep her busy with little girl versions of Girlology.

Girlology has become a recognized and welcomed program in the Southeast that is ripe for broad distribution. Girlology's focus on suburban girls and families serves an often neglected population that is overscheduled, undersupervised and frequently oversexed. Both Dr. Holmes and Dr. Hutchison are known for their rapport with teen girls and their liberal use of slang words for anything pertaining to sex or the human body. Their husbands can only hope that they censor their vocabulary in public, and their mothers keep wishing they would act like proper Southern girls.

For more information on Girlology programs, check out their Web site at *www.girlology.com.*

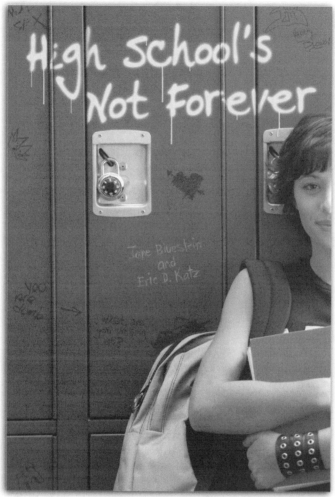

Code #2564 • $12.95

Your survival guide to the maze
that is the highschool experience.

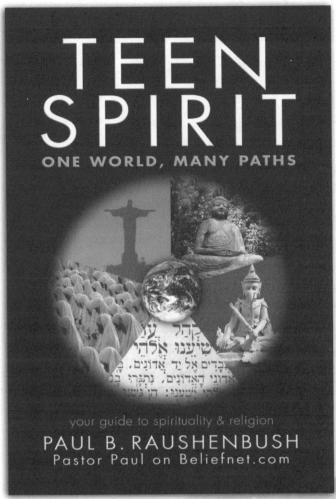

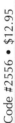
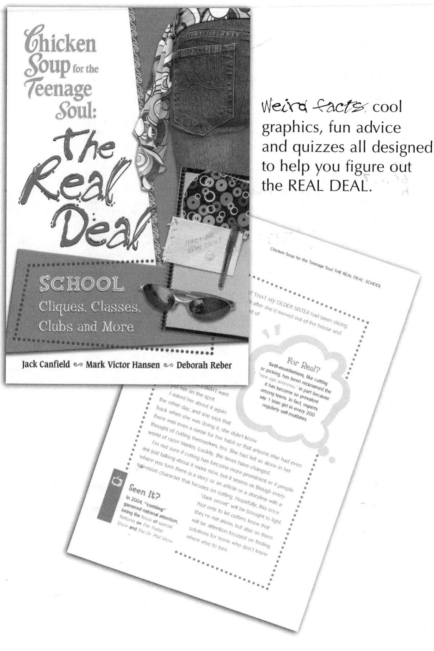